Calcium, Magnesium, and D3: Prevent and Eliminate Serious Illnesses

"Discover the Best Way to Use Ca, Mg, and D3 to Live Disease Free"

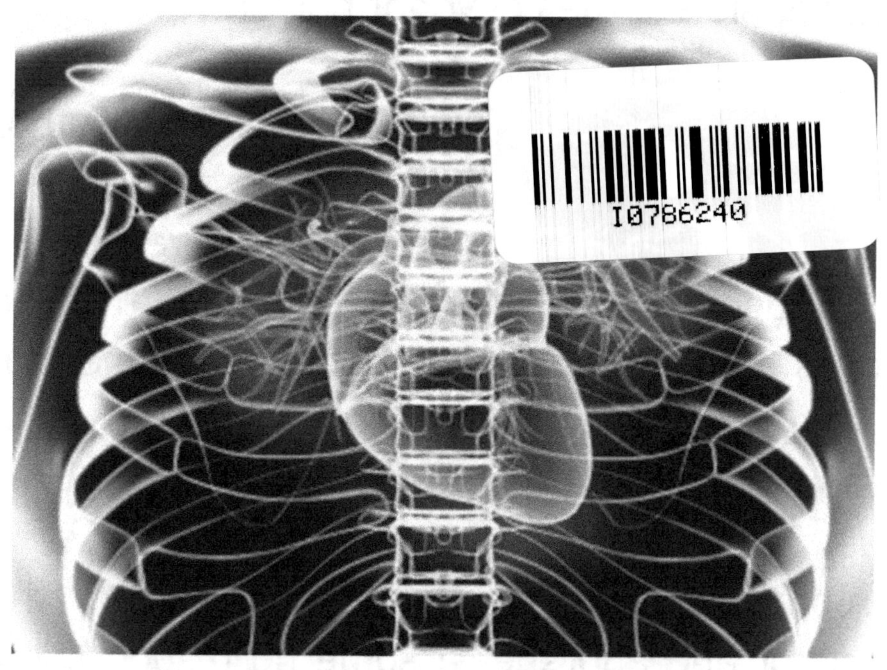

Rudy S Silva, Natural Nutritionist

How to Use Calcium, Magnesium, and Vitamin D3 to Prevent and Eliminate Illness, © 2013, New Edition 2018 by Rudy S Silva

Your doctor or health provider should confirm any information given here since it is not medical advice or treatment. This e-book is for information and educational purposes only. Consult with your doctor before using any of the remedies, recommendations, or information listed in this e-book.

First Printing, 2013, Second Printing, 2018, USA

TABLE OF CONTENTS

1: The 4 Most Important Nutrients To Use

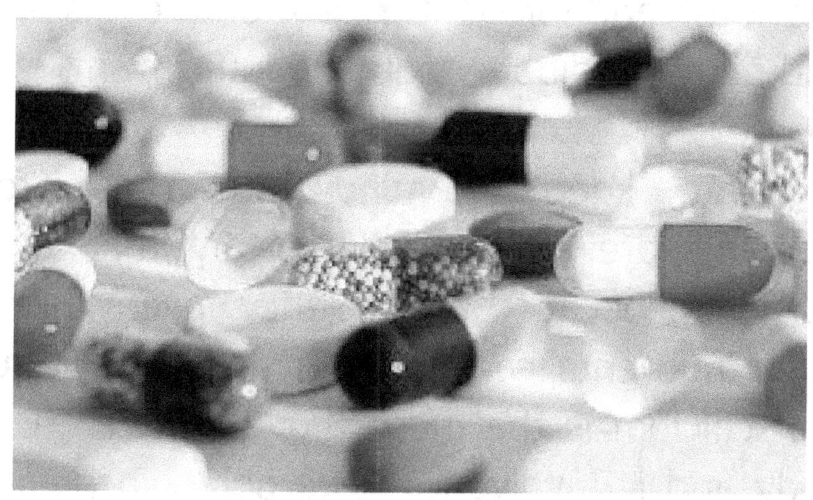

Calcium, Magnesium, D3, K2

Your body needs vitamin D3, K2, and magnesium to get calcium into your body. Without these three nutrients, you will absorb very little calcium and you will be plagued with various illnesses and you will die prematurely. Without magnesium, you can't activate the many benefits of vitamin D3. Once

This combination of these nutrients is probably one of the most important health concepts you need to get right. The power of vitamin D3 has the potential to diminish, alleviate, and prevent many of the diseases and body conditions that you suffer from.

But, keep in mind that these four nutrients are not more important than other nutrients, because a deficiency in any of the other nutrients can cause a disease. It just that calcium is the most active mineral in the body and is involved in the more biochemical reactions in your body than any other nutrient.

What is in This Book?

If you lack the body requirements of calcium, you will not be healthy. When you lack calcium, there are a number of illnesses your will contract. If you have too much calcium, this too will create poor health. This book will help you decide if you are deficient in calcium

In the following pages, you will discover how calcium, magnesium, vitamin D3, and vitamin K2 function in your body. You will find out what you need to do to make sure you are not deficient in these minerals.

Then, in the last chapter of this book, you will discover the power of vitamin D3 and vitamin K2 and how they must be used with calcium and magnesium. There are recommendations on how much of these nutrients you should be using as a group.

If you lack or have an excess of magnesium, this book will list the symptoms and diseases that you will be prone to. If you lack vitamin D, this book will help you discover how to maintain the proper levels of this vitamin. Vitamin D is the key to making sure you absorb calcium and magnesium into your blood.

The nutrients Calcium, magnesium, Vitamin K2 and vitamin D3, work together to get the most calcium into your blood and cells.

The Calcium Story

Calcium occurs in the earth as limestone, calcium carbonate, as gypsum, or as apatite. It is always found combined with other elements. You will never find a pure calcium rock.

When these types of calcium compounds combine with water, they dissolve and form an alkaline solution. This is one of the reasons why you want to know as much about calcium and use the right amount since it is one of the main elements that can make your body liquids alkaline.

One of the most important health programs you need to pursue is to move your body from an acid condition into an alkaline condition and calcium is the major mineral that helps you do this.

When your body is maintained consistently in an acid condition, calcium is also consistently removed from your bones, organs and lymph liquid. This results in porous bones, organ stones, organs degradation and cell degeneration.

Calcium is the most abundant minerals in your body and it makes up 1.6% of your body weight or represents 40% of all of the minerals in your body. But, 99% of the calcium you have is located in your bones. The other 1% is distributed throughout your body and is involved in numerous structural and biochemical processes.

Bone Loss

Bone loss starts around middle age. For women, it increases during menopause. For men, bone loss is slow, but steady starting from around 30. In bone loss, there are normally no symptoms. But, here are a few that stand out:

- Bone deformity or rickets

- Muscle and leg cramps

- Insomnia

- Growth retardation

Unfortunately, around 40% of women who live over 75 years will experience bone loss fractures. Here are some reasons for low bone mass at any age.

- Diet lacks the daily use of fruits and vegetables
- Lack of fiber
- Excess use of sodas
- Slender body or low weight
- Premature menopause
- Anorexia nervosa
- Extreme athletic training
- Lack of exercise or a sedentary lifestyle
- Excess eating or using various types of meat or protein, phosphorus, sodium, caffeine, wheat bran, and alcohol
- Smoking
- Use of corticosteroid or other medications
- Prolong bed rest or confined to a wheelchair

It has been found that if you lack a small drop in the required level of calcium in your body this deficiency will activate aging and many degenerative diseases. Even though calcium is a large atom, it chemically moves 10,000 times faster and is 10,000 times stronger than magnesium.

The King of the Bioelements

Magnesium gives calcium the ability to bind quickly and strongly with important biological molecules, which sustains life. This chemical's flexibility gives calcium the honor of being called "the King of the Bioelements."

In this book, you will discover why it has this name. Despite there is more calcium in the body than any other minerals, with exception of oxygen, calcium is not more important than the other minerals, since all work together and are needed in your body for maintaining life.

What we can say about calcium is that it

is involved in more biochemical activities in your body than any other mineral, so that it is important to supply your body with a good amount of calcium. Your body will eliminate the excess calcium from your body, even when it is in a supersaturated form in your body liquids.

But, when there is a deficiency of other minerals in your body that must balance with calcium, like sodium, excess calcium can react un-naturally, causing calcium crystalline deposits, which lead to pain and disease.

When your body lacks calcium and has weak or porous bones, calcium will deposit calcium crystalline stones in various places in your body as it tries to build up weak bones. A misconception is that if you have calcium deposits in the joints or tissue giving you pain, that you have too much calcium.

The truth is you do not have enough calcium, so the body tries to compensate for this by calcium deposits, to build your bones back up.

Sodium-Potassium Pump

Calcium is found in your blood, bone structure, tissue, muscles, lymph liquid, and in everybody cell in your body. It is found in the lymph liquid outside and inside your cells. In the so-called **Sodium-Potassium Pump,** the mineral sodium moves out of the cell and moves potassium into the cell. When the inside of the cell has mostly potassium, the electrical charge inside the cell is less than the charge outside of the cell where sodium dominates. This condition attracts calcium to carry nutrients into the cell and to perform various biochemical and bioelectrical reactions.

Calcium ions also play a major role in nerve stimulations and transmissions, muscle contractions and movements, and organ hormone secretions. It is involved with your body's enzymes to produce energy. It makes your body more alkaline, an important function to keep you disease free. Having excess acids in your cells leads to cell destruction.

Calcium ionic concentrations are the most regulated mineral in your blood plasma. Its ionic form is Ca^{++}. In this form, it's most important function is in nerve function. For nerve function, calcium keeps your nerves receptive to sodium ions, which transmit brain impulses and information to various parts of the body to regulate your body's activities.

In cultures, where drinking water had a high content of calcium, it was found that people's lifespan was 10 years or more than in western countries.

Kidneys

Your kidneys act as filters for your blood. They remove those nutrients or chemicals, from your blood, that your body no longer needs, including calcium. Excess calcium is routed to your bladder where it is expelled in your urine. If calcium is still needed, your kidneys pass it into your blood to be reused by your body.

Most minerals and vitamins combine and react with calcium to produce the various body structures and chemicals that make up your body.

It was thought at one time that if you produced kidney stones that you needed to take less calcium. If you tend to form kidney stones, you will have increased calcium in your urine, but this is caused by your body pulling calcium out of your bones.

Because eating excess meat causes your body to excrete calcium, it is recommended, for kidney stones, to eat less meat. Then, increase the use of fruits and vegetables, and supplement with calcium citrate, magnesium, vitamin D3, vitamin B6, and vitamin C.

You can take calcium citrate on an empty stomach. Most other supplements, you should take with meals.

Calcium Toxicity

Usually, there is no calcium toxicity, even when you take a large dose. Your body normally uses only 800 mg of calcium per day and it gets rids of the rest. If you take 2000 mg of calcium per day, your body may only absorb 20% of this supplement. The rest of it is excreted in your stools.

There is some concern that people with a tendency toward kidney stones should avoid excess calcium, but these concerns have not been proven. Kidney stones are more related to diet and those people who favor an acid diet tend to form kidney stones. In an acid diet, calcium is active and depleted as it is used up neutralizing body acids.

2: The Magic Of Calcium In Your Body

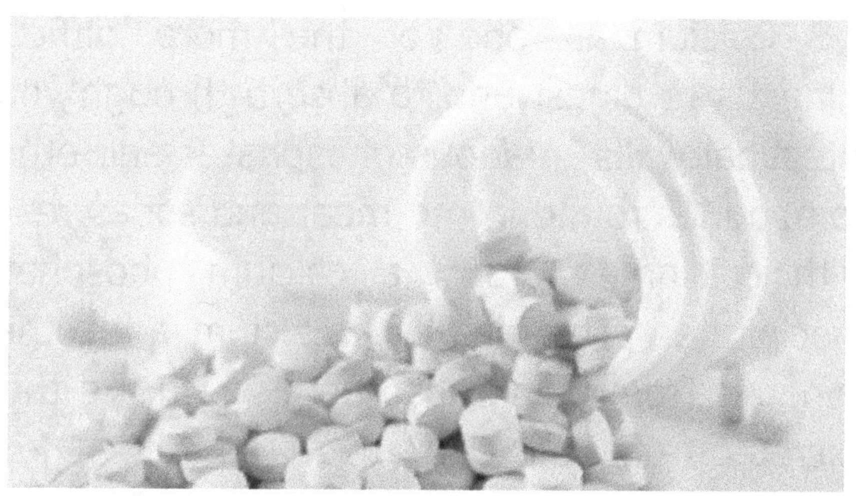

Functions of Calcium

Here is a list of some of the important biochemical and bioelectrical functions of calcium in the body:

- Activity in cell function
- Maintaining an alkaline body
- Contributing to Saliva alkaline body test
- Useful in preventing cancer
- Needed in DNA synthesis and cell division

- Will extend life
- Needed to prevent and treat disease

Adsorption of Calcium

Calcium is one of the more difficult minerals to digest and to absorb through your intestinal walls. Various phosphates and other compounds found in red meat and sodas react with calcium to form a calcium phosphate precipitate. This prevents calcium and other minerals from being absorbed, which are then excreted from your body.

(*Phosphates are derived from phosphoric acid and when it combines with oxygen it becomes an organic phosphate, which has important biochemical activities in your body*)

However, when calcium comes in contact with milk and various fruits and vegetables, it forms compounds that are easily absorbed.

For calcium to be absorbed into your body, it needs adequate vitamin D. Without

Vitamin D, calcium cannot pass through your intestines and into your bloodstream.

Vitamin D can be obtained from the sun and is critical in the amount of calcium absorption that occurs in your small intestine. This is why you need to get at least 30 minutes of sun every day. In some parts of the world less time is needed and in other parts more time is needed.

If you are dark-skinned, your skin produces less vitamin D than if you were light skinned. By being out in the sun, the amount of vitamin D that you can create depends on how much of your skin is exposed, the color of your skin, and how long you stay in the sun. Estimates have been made that you can form 10,000 to 100,000 IU of vitamin D every day in the sun.

You can also get vitamin D from supplements. Some foods have it but in very small quantities.

Inositol Triphosphate

When the sun's UV light hits your skin, fatty acids in your skin create vitamin D and **Inositol triphosphate, INSP-3**.   Then, vitamin D finds its way into your intestinal wall where it assists calcium to move through them and into your bloodstream.

Inositol triphosphate finds its way into every body cell.   Its function is to release calcium from storage from within your cells when insufficient calcium is not absorbed from food and supplements.

Inositol is obtained from foods such as fruits, vegetables, grains, and from liver, kidney, and heart.

Parathyroid Gland and Calcitonin

When there is insufficient calcium in the cell walls, because it got used up, the parathyroid hormone stimulated by a deficiency of vitamin D activates the extraction of calcium from your bones.   Once the bones become weaken, your body starts extracting calcium from proteins that regulate your cell functions. This results in a variety of aliment and disease symptoms.

Once in your bloodstream, calcium is deposited in bones with the help of the hormone, **calcitonin**, released by the parathyroid gland. Also, both Calcitonin and Inositol triphosphate regulate the storage and removal of calcium within the cells.

The parathyroid gland is regulated by the pituitary gland, which is right behind the eyes. When you wear sunglasses this blocks the full spectrum UV light that is needed to regulate the pituitary gland. Without this UV light, hormones needed to regulate calcium in your cells would not be possible.

Without adequate amounts of vitamin D, calcium will not be absorbed in proper amounts into your body and would be excreted from your body.

Parathyroid – How it regulates calcium

The parathyroid is actively involved in maintaining your calcium blood levels. These levels are maintained to a very strict range. When your blood calcium levels drop, the parathyroid releases a hormone that directs the release of calcium from your bones and into your bloodstream. And at the same time, it tells your kidneys not to excrete calcium into your urine.

Now, when you have excess calcium in your blood, the amount of the parathyroid hormone secreted is decreased. This causes the kidneys to expel more calcium into your urine. As all of this is happening, the parathyroid also releases a hormone called Calcitonin, which reduces the amount of calcium that is pull out of your bones.

Activity in Cell Function

Calcium is active in the Sodium-Potassium Pump process in that it uses this pump to enter and exit a cell. When it enters the cell, it brings in nutrients to feed the cell.

Once it releases these nutrients, it becomes a free calcium ion. As these calcium ions build up in the cell, the voltage across the cell membrane will again reach 70 millivolts. This sets the stage for nutrients and toxins in the cell to be pushed out of the cell and for other nutrients to enter the cell.

Maintaining an alkaline body

The fluid outside the cells is called extracellular fluid. This fluid is maintained at a pH of 7.4 by a calcium compound called calcium mono orthophosphate. This fluid is capable of neutralizing acids that come out of the cells or arrive there from food that you have eaten.

Sodium is also in the extracellular fluid and can neutralize acids, but it is needed in large quantities to maintain the Sodium-Potassium Pump cell activity. Wherever calcium is in the tissue, joints, blood, liquid or organs, it will neutralize acids. This process reduces damage to your tissues and elevates your body's pH, making it more alkaline.

When you don't have enough calcium in your body, the cells will not have enough calcium to neutralize body acids and this caused cell deterioration and diseases. Keeping your body liquids alkaline or with a pH above 6.8 to 7.4 is what you should be working towards in any health program. This can be done by using the right alkaline diet.

An alkaline diet helps you balance the level of acid and alkaline in all parts of your body. When you eat more acid foods, such as meat, butter, fats, carbohydrates, then your body will use up its alkaline stores to neutralize then acid residue created by these foods.

When you eat more alkaline foods than you need, you run the risk of not getting enough protein or carbohydrate and your pH can move above 7. 5 to 8.0. A high alkaline pH, 6.0 to 8.0 can also lead to disease. You need a balance of certain foods to get your body's pH in the range of 7.0

The saliva alkaline body test

In the kindle book called "Alkaline Body," the saliva test has been discussed in greater detail. This test is a strong indicator of whether your calcium ion level is sufficient.

Here is a review

You can measure the saliva in your mouth and get a fairly accurate measure of the pH in your body. Saliva is created in your body and is brought into your mouth through two saliva glands. Your body produces gallons of saliva every day, so measuring your saliva is a good indicator of what is happening inside your body.

Wait at least a couple of hours after you eat to do this saliva test. When you start, bring saliva 3 times into your mouth and swallow. On the 4th time, wet a strip of pH paper in your mouth and pull it out. Now, you can read it.

(Purchase some pH litmus paper at a drug store, laboratory outlet or order it through the Internet. The better pH paper you can buy comes in .25 increments in pH change. You can buy this litmus paper on Amazon.)

When your Saliva pH is 6.8 to 7.4 it is considered alkaline and normal. When this is the case, your urine will be slightly acidic and in the range of 5.5 to 6.5. When you lack ionic calcium, your saliva pH will be 4.6 to 6.4 and your urine will even more acidic.

Now here is important information on your saliva test.

If you have physical ailments, your pH will be from 6.0 to 6.7. In this case, you should take around 2000 mg of calcium rather than 1000 mg.

If your pH is below 5.0 to 6.0, most likely, you will have various disease symptoms.

And, you should be taking around 3000 mg of calcium. Once you bring up your salivary pH, you can lower your calcium intake.

If your saliva tests show your pH to be below 6.0, then by taking more calcium supplements and by eating more fruits and vegetable during the day and especially in the evening, you can change your pH to 6.8 to 7.4.

Keep in mind that the saliva test may not always be accurate since the saliva pH can be influenced by food recently eaten. To get the most accurate reading, take the saliva test 2 hours after eating your last meal or snack. Take the test 3 times on 3 different days to make sure your readings are consistent. In my kindle e-book called "Alkaline Body," it shows you how you can change your body from 6.0 to 7.4 pH.

Simply by changing your diet, taking vitamins, and mineral supplements when you eat, you can change your body's pH to the 7.0 to 7.4 level. When you do this, you will see a change in any physical ailment and disease that you might have. It will not occur instantly. You will need to keep this pH level for a few months.

In the past, it was said that you did not need to take supplements. You could get all the nutrition your body needed from the food you ate. Today is a different story. The food supply lacks nutrients and most food in the grocery store is processed and junk food. And, it is necessary to supplement your diet with supplements or expect to develop some form of illness.

Another Saliva Tes

Here is another way to approach your saliva test. This was outlined in my Alkaline Body book.

Saliva Test

Here is a simple test you can perform on your saliva that will give you an idea of where you stand with your body's pH level. Your saliva contains mineral salts that keep it alkaline at 6.8 to 7.4. If your body is deficient in alkaline food or minerals, it will take the minerals from your saliva causing it to drop in pH.

If your saliva is below normal, you can influence your saliva's pH to read higher, by eating more acid binding (acid binding food will be explained in the next chapter) food and by supplementing with potassium, magnesium, and calcium.

Keep in mind there are some inaccuracies with this method since your body fluids are always in transition. This test simply gives you an idea of what your saliva pH is at that moment.   Use this information for your own education.   Then as you begin to change your eating habits and lifestyle, you can retest to see if there is a difference.

Many doctors deny the accuracy or use of this saliva test and say it is of no value. Frankly, they prefer you to pay them a visit, so that they can put you under their care.

In an article written by Dr. Steven Zodkoy, A Free and Simple Test for pH, a Potential Health Tester, Dr. Zodkoy recommends using the saliva pH test to determine the state of your body's pH.

By testing your pH regularly, you can decide the validity of using pH litmus paper to determine the level of your health. As you make changes, you can test your saliva and urine to see if the pH litmus color changes.

You need to take this test for 3 days and at least 3 times a day and to get an average value so you can establish a baseline or a starting point for yourself.

Purchase some pH litmus paper at a drug store, laboratory outlet or order it through the Internet. The better pH paper you can buy it on the internet, with a .25 increment in pH change. Purchase the type that is test strips and not in roll form.

Starting Your Saliva Testing

Gather saliva in your mouth then swallow. Do this three times.

Place the pH paper under your tongue. Let it sit there for 5 seconds to wet it and then remove it. Let it sit for 10 to 20 seconds, compare the color of your pH paper to the color chart on the bottle and record the pH.

Do this test around one hour before eating or around two hours after eating. This reading gives you an idea about the state of your saliva. Your first test should be done first thing in the morning before you rinse out your mouth or drink anything.

Saliva and Lemon Test

Now, do this test immediately after you do your saliva test above. Squeeze the juice of half a lemon into one ounce of water, and swish it around in your mouth for 5 seconds or so. Then spit it out, wait one minute, now, measure your mouth's pH with litmus paper.

Just place the paper into your mouth and wet it.

Now compare the color and pH value of this reading with your first pH saliva reading. This reading should have a higher alkaline reading than your first saliva reading.

Good Saliva Test

Reading, it means you have alkaline reserves. The higher the alkaline reading you have the stronger your alkaline reserves. A small alkaline upward change means you have alkaline reserves If this reading has a higher alkaline, but they are not as strong as they should be.

For example,

- Morning reading is 6.5 pH

- After the lemon test reading 6.9 pH

These readings are good and indicate you have some alkaline mineral stores. But, your Morning reading of 6.5 is a little low and should be closer to 6.8 to 7.0 for better health.

Weak Saliva Test

If your pH reading does not change from your first reading or actually goes down, by becoming more acidic, then your alkaline reserves are weak. You need to make some major changes in the way you eat. In this course, you will see what you need to do to bring up your alkaline reserves so that you will not be susceptible to serious diseases.

Now, suppose your readings were,

First reading 6.5

Lemon test reading 6.2

There is a drop in your lemon pH test, and this is not good. This means that you don't have enough minerals in your body to neutralize the acid in your mouth. You will have to eat more acid binding food.

Saliva Test Summary

Again, if your lemon test readings have a higher pH reading than your first reading, it means you have alkaline reserves. The bigger the difference between your first test and second test, the stronger your alkaline reserves. A small alkaline upward change means you have alkaline reserves, but they are not as strong as they should be.

If your lemon pH reading does not change from your first reading or actually goes down by becoming more acidic, then your alkaline reserves are weak, and you need to make some major changes in the way you eat. This also means you have a highly acidic body that can create some serious illness, especially if your lemon test pH is down to 6.0 and below.

3: Illnesses Caused by Lack of Calcium

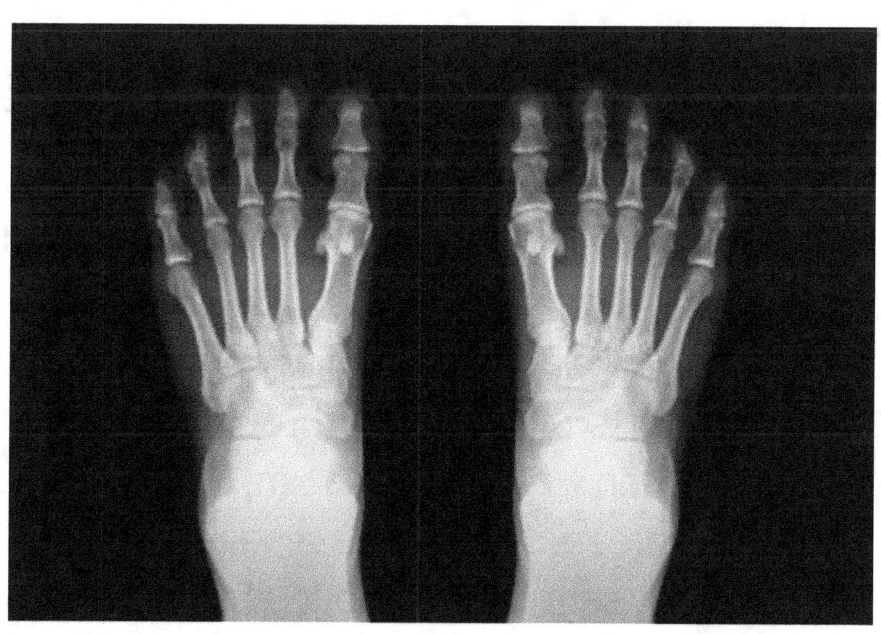

What Calcium Does in Your Body

Calcium plays a major role in blood, cells, liver, kidney, bone, muscles, and heart health. Calcium maintains blood pH to 7.4, solidifies bones, and helps heal scars, and fights scurvy and germs. It is present in cartilage, fluids, and tissue. It is useful for Indigestion, headaches, muscle pains, arthritis, ileitis, colitis, and asthma.

Calcium is now considered necessary to prevent cancer and should be used when you have it. The one thing to remember is calcium from food sources does not contribute to arteriosclerosis, calcium deposits, increase blood pressure, and other illnesses.

Calcium is one of the main minerals that promote healing in bones, tissue, organs, brain and in all parts of the body. It is carried to various parts of the body through the blood vessels. When you lack calcium, the infected or weaken areas do not get repaired properly and disease sets in. Without the necessary calcium your body needs, blood coagulation is affected and excess bleeding can occur.

Sun Glasses

Sunlight is a necessary energy that helps to ensure the absorptions of calcium through vitamin D. But, sunlight also plays another important role in regulating calcium in your body.

Sunlight or full spectrum white light plays a major role in how the pituitary and pineal glands work. In the workplace, however, the lighting is artificial and this has a big impact on your long-term health.

The use of sunglasses is quite popular and because of the many different sunglass tints that exist, people wearing them to filter out the sunlight frequencies associated with that tint.

In his book, The Calcium Factor: The Scientific Secret of Health and Youth, 2000, Robert R. Barefoot & Carl J. Reich, M.D. says,

"When artificial full spectrum lighting is used, human calcium absorption increases, plants flourish and cows produce 15% more milk...Tinted glasses can eliminate a large percentage of the sun's spectrum and therefore affect you both physically and psychologically. Thus, full spectrum light plays a vital role in the maintenance of a balanced hormonal system and is therefore indispensable in maintaining a balanced calcium serum."

Osteoporosis

Osteoporosis is the lack of calcium in the bones and it is estimated that over 30% of the older population will develop this condition. This lack causes bones to become porous, brittle, and weak and more susceptible to breakage. This is not a condition that results from old age, but a condition that comes from having an acid body for a long time.

Since the endocrine glands exert a great amount of control over calcium, the endocrine glands are put out of balance by sugar. This causes an imbalance in calcium, which shows up as cavities in your teeth.

It is the imbalance of calcium in your body that is the start of the development of chronic illnesses.

Menstrual Flow

Menstrual blood contains up to 40 times more calcium than regular blood. If you have excessive flow, then you become depleted of calcium and iron. During this period, you should be eating kale, using liquid chlorophyll, and the many foods outlined in these chapters.

Without using a program that replaces your loss of calcium and iron during your periods, you open yourself to various diseases later on. For a diet that contains plenty of iron, you can check out my e-book called, "Quick and Easy Diet Cures 4 Iron Deficiency Anemia."

Teeth health

Your teeth are made up of calcium phosphate. They are kept healthy by your blood and the nutrients that you supply them. The external part of your teeth is protected by enamel, which is an extremely strong material. But, acids that form in your mouth, when sugar is eaten, it creates an excess of bacteria that can penetrate that enamel.

Having dental cavities is a sign of a lack of calcium. When your body needs calcium and you have not provided enough in your diet, calcium is pulled out of your teeth and bones to bring your body back into calcium balance. This weakens your teeth and bacteria can penetrate the enamel causing tooth decay.

Arteriosclerosis

Arteriosclerosis is not caused by an excess of calcium. It is caused by the lack of sodium and chlorine salts. Calcium needs these salts to be properly used and to stay in solution and not precipitate out onto artery walls. It is needed so that artery walls don't become inflamed by acid damage and free radicals. When damaged arteries need repair through cholesterol and plaque buildup.

Arteriosclerosis occurs when plaque builds up along the artery walls, which takes place over years. Eventually, this plaque will narrow the arteries and cause reduced blood flow or blood flow blockage. Reduced blood flow will result in many different illnesses because your organs and cells will not be getting the proper oxygen and nutrition. Artery blockage will result in heart attacks.

Plaque is made up of phospholipids, collagen, triglycerides, fibrin, mucopolysaccharides, cholesterol, heavy metals, proteins, muscle tissue, and debris, which are all bonded by calcium.

Plaque only occurs in arteries that deliver blood from the heart to your body and not in the veins that return blood to the heart. Cholesterol is not the cause of plaque, but even if it was, it can be controlled by diet and not drugs.

Eighty percent of the cholesterol in your body is created in the body and 20% of it comes from your diet. Your body uses cholesterol in every cell, in hormones, in nerve impulses, in the brain, and in the creation of vitamin D on your skin.

Heart Disease

Calcium is central to good heart function. Since calcium ions are linked to proper cell function, any lack of calcium can affect heart cell function. This lack of calcium can lead to heart diseases over a long time. The ability of your heart to contract and expand is due to the ionization of calcium, Ca++, in your heart cells.

Effects of Excess Calcium

When your body has an excess of calcium, you will see external and internal boney growths. These growths can occur in any part of your body, such as joints, tissue, organs, or muscle. The growths may appear as kidney stones or other precipitates that occur on your heels, shoulder joints, knee joints, or toe bones.

When you have excess calcium, you need to eat more fruits and vegetables to get the natural absorbable vitamins and minerals, especially sodium and magnesium. Calcium, Sodium, magnesium must always be in balance. Lacking one or the other leads to a chemical imbalance, which results in various illnesses or diseases.

Calcium and magnesium need to be in a certain balance to prevent lack of blood calcium. Studies have shown that it is best to have a calcium to magnesium ratio of 1:1. Past recommendations have been a 2:1 ratio.

When you have high calcium to magnesium, 4:1 ratio, you are more susceptible to heart attacks. Although plenty of calcium is recommended, so is plenty of magnesium.

Illness or Conditions Due To Lack of Calcium

Here some of the symptoms or conditions that occur when you lack calcium:

- tumors
- sores, abscesses, inflammations
- discharges
- deformed fingers, bones, hips cranial bones
- tooth decay
- undersized organs
- blood deficiencies
- back pain
- vomiting
- tuberculosis
- excess bleeding
- excess mucus discharge
- poor scar healing
- craving for salt
- bone softening
- swelling knuckles
- bronchial congestion
- wrinkled skin
- cystic goiter
- cyst formation
- nervous problems

There are so many illness and poor body conditions that occur when you lack calcium.

You may have a few of these, but if they are consistent and they remain with you for a while, consider taking more calcium with magnesium.

Nervous Problems

Anxiety is supposed to help you when you are involved in stressful or life threating situation.   Under these conditions your metabolism increases, muscles tighten, and you get a shot of adrenaline. When anxiety happens, you use up many minerals, including calcium.   Under stressful conditions that last more than a day, it is wise to take a calcium supplement.

Back pain

Back pain is one of those conditions that when it occurs, it can disable you and cause you to take a quick trip to the emergency. When back pain is caused by strained muscles, stress, bad posture, inactivity, or lack of exercise, one of the supplements recommend is calcium with magnesium. These minerals reduce muscle spasms, muscle tightness, and nerve irritation.

Taking a supplement that contains calcium, magnesium, vitamin D3, and K2 daily, will help you to alleviate the long list of body conditions or illnesses. Just remember that calcium is a relaxer and nerve reliever.

4: The Best Calcium Foods to Eat

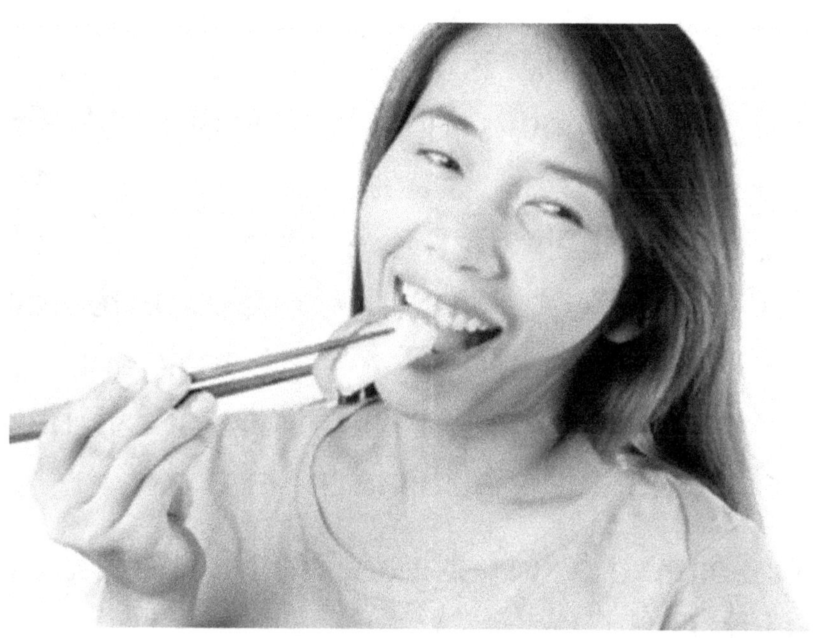

Calcium absorption

Even though you eat calcium foods, only around 25% of the calcium in this food will be absorbed by your body. But, as a child or if you are pregnant, you may absorb up to 60%.

When cooking fruits or vegetables, you should use lower temperatures, when possible. When produce is heated above 150 Fahrenheit at least 33% of the available calcium is lost.

Calcium and Milk

All milk that is pasteurized at high temperature is a low source of calcium. There is some milk that is pasteurized at 145 degrees Fahrenheit that is a better source of calcium. All milk that has been pasteurized or homogenized is acidic. The best milk source for calcium is raw goat milk, and since it has not been heated it is alkaline in nature.

Despite the insistence from The Dairy Council that,

"Milk has been part of the diet for thousands of years. Despite the fact that milk is one of the most nutritionally complete foods available, there are many myths relating to its consumption that blame milk and dairy foods for a variety of ailments. Many of these myths have been part of the folklore for centuries and are not founded on science."

There is a tremendous amount of scientific papers and findings that milk should not be included in your diet, because of the illnesses it contributes too. But, then again there are studies that show there is a decrease in heart and cancer in people that drink milk. Just remember milk is an acid food and has to be balanced off with alkaline food.

An article, In 1992 The New England Journal of Medicine pointed out that, "Consumption of cow's milk has been associated with insulin-dependent diabetes..."

There are other sources of dairy products that can provide plenty of calcium for your diet, such as unsweetened yogurt or cottage cheese. To improve your calcium intake, eat plenty of those vegetables and fruits that are high in calcium.

In his book, **Prescription for Natural Cures**, 2004, by James F. Balch, M.D. he says,

"It may surprise you to learn that countries, where people drink the most milk, are also those with the highest rates of osteoporosis. This may be due to the fact that lactose intolerance and casein allergy are very common and lead to malabsorption. Also, calcium from cow's milk is not well absorbed, at a rate of 25 percent. Milk products lead to other health problems as well, so don't rely on them as a source of calcium. Unsweetened, cultured yogurt is an exception."

One way to eat your unsweetened yogurt is to put it in a blender, then add fruits like strawberries, pineapple, mango, bananas, or fruits you like. To get additional sweetness, you can add a small amount of raw honey, since honey will help you to absorb calcium.

The British Medical Research Council made a 10-year study of 5000 men aged 45 to 59. In this study, they found, "only 1 percent of those who regularly drank more than one-half liter of milk a day suffered heart attacks … against 10 percent of those who drank no milk at all." In this study, researchers also found there was no difference whether they drank pure milk or skimmed, the benefits were still there.

There is still a lot of controversy about drinking milk for calcium. If you feel good drinking milk, then you should drink it. If you develop mucus or other symptoms, when you drink milk, then you should consider getting your calcium from other sources.

Where you can get calcium

One of the highest sources of calcium comes from **barley, green kale,** and **turnip greens**. You can get good calcium from cereals and grains.

Here is a list of foods highest in calcium:

- Seaweed – dulse, kelp, Irish moss, wakame, nori, kombu, agar
- Sardines with bones
- Tempeh, tofu
- Avocados, figs, prunes

- All dark greens, collard greens, spinach, kale,
- Unprocessed seeds and nuts – sesame seeds, grains, and nuts, almonds, walnuts
- Bone Broth
- Cow and goat milk, cheese, cottage cheese, and yogurt
- Rice milk-calcium enriched
- Cabbage, cauliflower, celery, lemons, rhubarb
- Egg yolk, gelatin foods
- Fish, meat near the bone
- Whole wheat bread
- Beans, brown rice, lentils, millet, oats,
- Broccoli, Brussels sprouts, cauliflower
- Onions, parsnips, watercress
- Raw butter, gelatin, blackstrap molasses
- Coconut, raw cream, egg yolk
- Fish, meat near the bone, bone broth
- Natural cane sugar

The amount of calcium in certain foods

½ cup of wakame – sea vegetable gives 1700 mg

¼ cup of agar – sea vegetable gives 1000 mg

½ cup of nori – sea vegetable gives 600 mg

¼ cup of kombu – sea vegetable gives 500 mg

1 cup of tempeh gives 340 mg

8 oz. of calcium enriched rice milk give 300 mg.

1 cup of almonds gives 300 mg

8 oz. of skim milk gives 302 mg

8 oz. of low-fat yogurt gives 300 mg

1 oz. of Swiss cheese gives 272 mg

10 figs give 269 mg

½ cup of tofu gives 258 mg

½ cup of sesame seeds gives 250 mg

1 oz. of mozzarella cheese gives 183 mg

½ cup of boiled collards gives 179 mg

1 tablespoon of blackstrap molasses gives 172 mg

1 cup cottage cheese gives 126 mg

2 sardines in oil give 92 mg

¼ cup of walnuts gives 70 mg

1 cup of black beans or lentils give 55 mg

½ cup of boiled mustard greens gives 52 mg

½ cup of boiled broccoli gives 36 mg

Dark Greens

The dark greens can be boiled instead of steamed and their taste is improved. Boiling them also does not cause them to reduce their nutritional value since they have such high nutrition, to begin with.

Meat

Limit the amount of meat you eat. Meat has 30 times more phosphorous than calcium. And, in the digestive tract, this phosphorous will cause the calcium to precipitate to form apatite, which is a form of a phosphorous calcium mineral crystal. It is apatite that is the substance that forms your bones. The result is that this calcium is not available to you and is excreted from your body.

Sugar

It has been found that there is 40% less calcium in white sugar as compared to raw sugar. Blackstrap molasses has 258 times more calcium as white sugar. Calcium and sugar attract each other. The more sugar you eat the more calcium is precipitated. The less body calcium you have the more tooth decay you will have.

Salt

Using excess salt in your food has been associated with bone loss. If you eat salt with your food, salt competes with calcium to get absorbed. The more salt is absorbed the less calcium is.

Try using culinary herbs and chili sauces to flavor your food. If you like salty food, you could use them as a snack and not with your regular meals.

Nightshades

Foods like tomatoes, potatoes, eggplant, peppers, and tobacco are considered nightshade foods.

In her book, Food and Healing, 1986, Annemarie Colbin pointed out that,

"In my own experience and that of some of my students, consuming nightshades on a dairy-free diet has resulted in a loss of calcium, evidenced by brittle nails, painful gums, and dental caries. Eliminating the nightshades, rather than increasing the dairy, solved the problem"

There are some foods that promote the excretion of calcium. We have indicated that eating excess meat can trap calcium and eliminate it from your body.

Oxalic and Phytic Acid

Foods high in oxalic acid also promote the removal of calcium from your body – spinach, cranberries, and rhubarb.

Wheat bran also limits the amount of calcium you absorb, because of the phytic acid in its fiber. The phytic acid in wheat fiber has the ability to combine with calcium and limit its absorption in your body.

Other things that limit your calcium absorption are eating too many foods that contain phosphorus, drinking tea which contains tannins, lack of vitamin D, and having diarrhea.

Pumpkin Seeds

Shelled pumpkin seeds are a high source of zinc, magnesium, iron, phosphorus, and calcium. Eat a hand full every day.

5: Calcium Supplements You Must Take

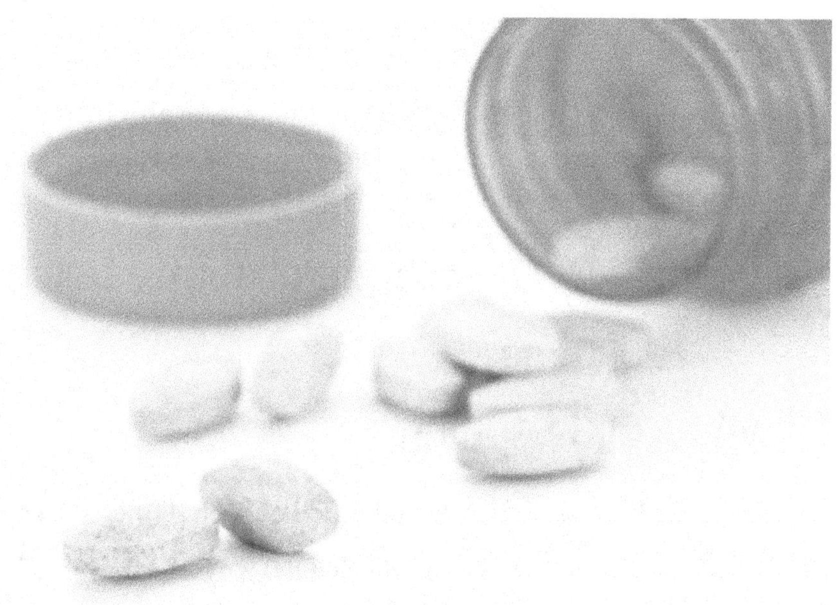

Calcium Supplements

Taking calcium supplements is a great idea since you are probably not getting all of the calcium you need in your diet.

However, since calcium tends to interfere with the absorption of other minerals, it is best to also take a multivitamin that provides those other minerals.

What type of calcium supplements should you take? A good supplement is one that contains:

Calcium 1000 – 1500 mg

Magnesium 400 – 600 mg

Vitamin D Cholecalciferol form, called D3, 1000 mg

Vitamin K2, 100 ng

So what are your daily requirements for calcium? Daily requirements for calcium are between 1000 to 1500mg. The type of supplement and the amount you take depends on your ability to absorb calcium. This is difficult to determine, so it is best to take the high end of calcium – 1500+ mg.

Here are some minimum calcium supplementation requirements. Keep in mind that if you can get this amount in your food then you don't need to take calcium supplements.

- Infants 7-12 months   270 mg
- Children 4-8 years   800 mg
- Males 31-50   1000 mg
- Females 31-50   1000 mg
- Pregnant and lactating   1000 mcg

One of the best calcium supplements to use is Brazil Live Coral. It contains calcium, vitamin D, magnesium, and all of the trace minerals. It is in powder form so it is more absorbable. It contains the vitamin D you need to absorb more calcium.

But, you also need to spend at least 20 to 30 minutes in the sun to get natural vitamin D. It does not have to be in the direct sunlight, but it is better if it is.

Look for **Brazil Live Coral** and for **Okinawa coral calcium** on the internet. Another excellent calcium supplement is called, **3-Way Calcium Complex™**. Look for this also on the internet. It uses three different forms of calcium and includes other nutrients that help you absorb more of the calcium.

Calcium absorption

For calcium to be absorbed into your body, it is crucial to have adequate vitamin D3 in your body. Without Vitamin D3, calcium cannot be absorbed into your body. Vitamin D3 can be obtained from the sun or from supplements. Be aware that wearing sunglasses can affect your health by not keeping your pituitary gland healthy.

It's the pituitary gland that tells the parathyroid to release hormones that help regulate and absorb calcium. In addition to eating calcium foods, take Brazil Live Coral Calcium and also add vitamin D as a supplement to your diet, especially if you don't go out into the sun every day.

Vitamin C

It is believed that by taking vitamin C with Calcium, you increase the absorption of calcium. A form of calcium that is already combined with vitamin C is called Calcium Ascorbate. This type of calcium is easily transported across the intestinal walls.

Chelated calcium

It is best to use calcium supplements in chelated form. What this means is that calcium is tied to an amino acid and this makes it easier for calcium to pass through your intestinal walls. Chelated calcium is more easily absorbed than calcium that is not chelated. Here are some of the types of calcium amino acid chelates you should look for and buy.

- Calcium Alpha Keto Gluconate
- Calcium ascorbate – a form of calcium that is tied to vitamin C
- Calcium Lactate
- Calcium Alginate
- Calcium hydroxyapatite – the type of calcium found in your bones
- Calcium Glycinate
- Calcium Amino Acid Chelate

- Calcium Caprylate
- Calcium Malate
- Calcium Gluconate
- Calcium L-Aspartate
- Calcium Lactate Gluconate
- Calcium Lysinate
- Calcium Orotate
- Calcium Succinate
- Tricalcium phosphate – the type of calcium in your bones

All of these amino acids tied to calcium can also be attached to other minerals like magnesium and potassium. So you can find magnesium alginate or magnesium alginate or magnesium aspartate.

Honey

It has been found by the United States Department of Agriculture nutritionist Richard J. Wood that the glucose in honey can increase your absorption of calcium by up to 25%. It can also increase the absorption of zinc and magnesium.

Types of Calcium to Avoid

Calcium Dolomite

Avoid using dolomite as a source of calcium, since it may not be absorbed properly by your body. Dolomite is a form of calcium carbonate and magnesium.

Calcium carbonate

Calcium carbonate is hard to absorb when the pH in your stomach is not at the proper level. The pH in your stomach will change if you are taking OTC reflux acid pills.

Magnesium

Magnesium is usually found in calcium supplements because it is required for proper calcium metabolism. Magnesium has a role in the formation of bones. It has been found that when there is a decrease in blood magnesium that there is also a drop in blood calcium. The lack of magnesium in your body can increase the risk of osteoporosis.

Magnesium's absorption is enhanced by vitamin D just as calcium is. Magnesium is active in making sure that cells function properly by moving sodium and potassium in and out of the cells. Magnesium, just like calcium, is important for nerve and heart function. Many of the foods that are high in calcium are also high in magnesium.

6: Why Calcium Will Make You Alkaline

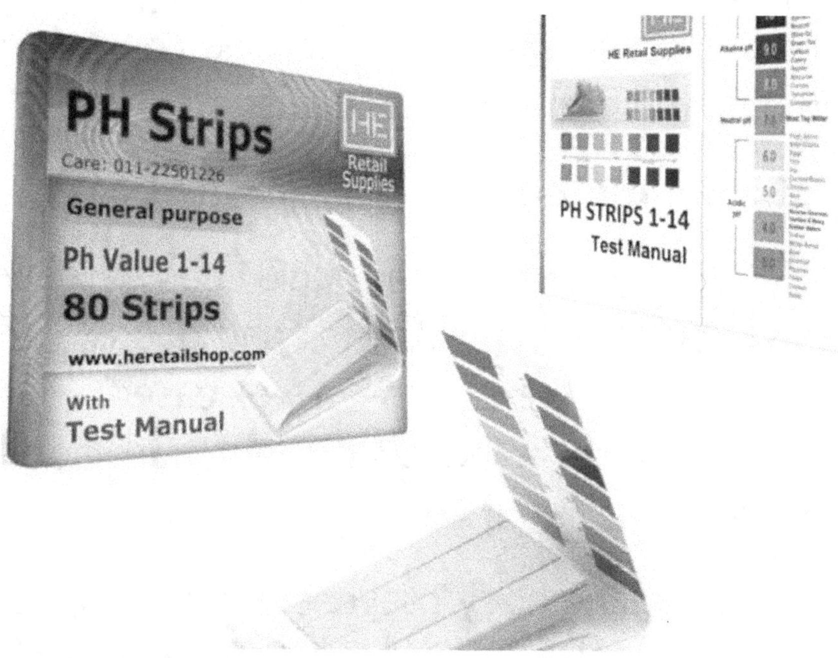

In this chapter, you will discover how you can make your body more alkaline. Calcium in addition to other minerals is one of the main minerals that can help you do this. Keeping your body alkaline is one of the best ways to keep your body calcium levels in balance.

Minerals

Making your body more alkalinity is what will help you gain better health. It is the minerals that strengthen your muscles and bones. They are necessary for the contraction and function of muscles and tissue.

Acid-Alkaline Body

When you have an acid body, it will attract disease. It attracts pathogens, and water, which produces a diseased body associated with being overweight and lacking the proper nutrition.

An alkaline body prevents your body from becoming ill and forming deadly diseases, like stomach problems, joint problems, organ degradation, body pain, heart disease, or even cancer. If you are already sick, then all of the chemicals inside fruits and vegetables will help to revive you to better health. This is provided that your tissue damage has not gone beyond repair.

The minerals most important in changing and maintaining your body in an alkaline condition are sodium, potassium, chloride, calcium, phosphorus, magnesium, and sulfur.

Now, how your body can become alkaline might become a little confusing at first because of the terms used.

Acid Binding

There are certain minerals that are called acid binding. And, these are minerals we said are the most important ones in fruits and vegetables - Sodium, potassium, calcium, phosphorus, and magnesium.

What acid binding means is when you eat produce with these minerals and various chemicals, the chemicals react in your cells to create energy. This reaction in your cells produces an alkaline residue. It is this residue that combines with acids in your body and neutralizes them. These neutralized acids are then eliminated from your body through your lungs, kidney, and colon.

If not all the acid toxins are captured by acid binding matter, the remaining acids can be neutralized by your body stores of alkaline minerals. If you don't have a good store of alkaline minerals, then these acids will remain in your body weakening it and creating disease. But, if you do have a good store of alkaline minerals, these minerals will find acids, capture them, bind with them, and eliminate them.

So you can see the importance of getting a lot of alkaline minerals into your body. Without them, acids would not get eliminated from your body, and they would remain in your body tissue and continue their body damage.

Alkaline Binding

Now, there are also minerals that become **alkaline binding** instead of **acid binding** and these minerals are sulfur, chlorine, iodine, phosphorus, bromine, fluorine, copper, and silicon. It is these minerals that when digested by a cell will produce a salt that will bind with alkaline minerals. These trapped alkaline binding salts will be excreted through your urine and other elimination channels.

When alkaline minerals are trapped by an acid salt, the alkaline minerals are removed from your body and your body becomes more acidic. This is the condition you are trying to avoid.

Foods that are alkaline binding and remove the minerals that you need to make your body alkaline are meat, carbohydrates, some vegetables and some fruits.

Although you need to eat both foods that are acid binding or alkaline binding, you want to eat more of the acid-binding foods. This will keep your body slightly alkaline.

Where do Acid Toxins Come From?

So why is the body overloaded with acid toxins?

Why can't the liver take care of all these toxins? Your liver has the function to remove acid wastes from food that is digestion and from cell metabolism. When your body encounters acid wastes, such as food enhancers, dyes, preservatives, pesticides, and the variety of food additives, the liver does not always know how to break them down or make them harmless.

Acid waste can also be created in your stomach. These are residues from incomplete digestion. As this waste, passes into your small intestine, they can be absorbed, if your intestinal walls suffer from leaky gut syndrome, conditions where large molecules are allowed to pass through the intestine wall. This acid waste then flows into the liver.

When your liver can't neutralize all acid

waste, it instructs calcium to bind with these toxic acids and to take them far away from the bloodstream.

Stress Creates Acids

Now, we have talked about acid toxins in the body that are brought in through food and the environment. But, there is another factor that creates acid waste in the body. Emotional problems create acidic molecules that embed themselves into your tissues just like food acids. These, again, can be removed with acid binding minerals.

Body Organs

All body organs, including your stomach, function to rid the body of acid waste or toxins. Lack of acid-binding food causes the deterioration of these organs. Each organ has a specific function in the elimination and neutralization of acid wastes and it does this in conjunction with acid binding minerals.

Acid Binding Foods

Here is a list of the fruits, and vegetables that have the highest alkaline minerals and that you should be eating to eliminate your body acids.

The percentage assigned to these fruits is based on fresh fruits that are organic, not cooked, canned or mixed with sugar. If they are cooked or otherwise processed in some fashion, this will reduce their effectiveness as an acid binding fruit. However, they will still be somewhat effective in acid binding.

Here is the list of fruits to eat in the order of priority.

1. **Fruits at 100% Acid Binding – Best fruits To Eat** Lemons, melons – any type, watermelon

2. **Fruits at 93% Acid Binding – Great fruits To Eat**

Cantaloupes, dried dates, dried figs, limes, mango, papaya

3. **Fruits at 87% Acid Binding – Still Great Fruits To Eat** Kiwis, passion fruit, pineapples, raisins, umeboshi plums

4. **Fruits at 80% Acid Binding – Eat These Fruits** Apricots, avocados, bananas, fresh dates, fresh figs, currants, gooseberries grapes, grapefruits guavas, kumquats, nectarines, pears, persimmons, quince

5. **Fruits at 73% Acid Binding – Still Fruits To Eat** Apples, organs, peaches, pomegranate, raspberries, sour grapes, strawberries

6. **Fruits at 67% Acid Binding** – Still Neutralizes Acids Cherries

Fruits to Concentrate On

These are the fruits you should concentrate on eating. Eat them every day. Drink fresh lemon juice in the morning and watermelon during the day.

You can see which fruits give you the best acid binding effects. Eat them most of the time, until your body becomes more alkaline.

NOW LET'S GO TO THE NEXT SECTION
ON
MAGNESIUM

7: Why Magnesium is Critical for Your Health

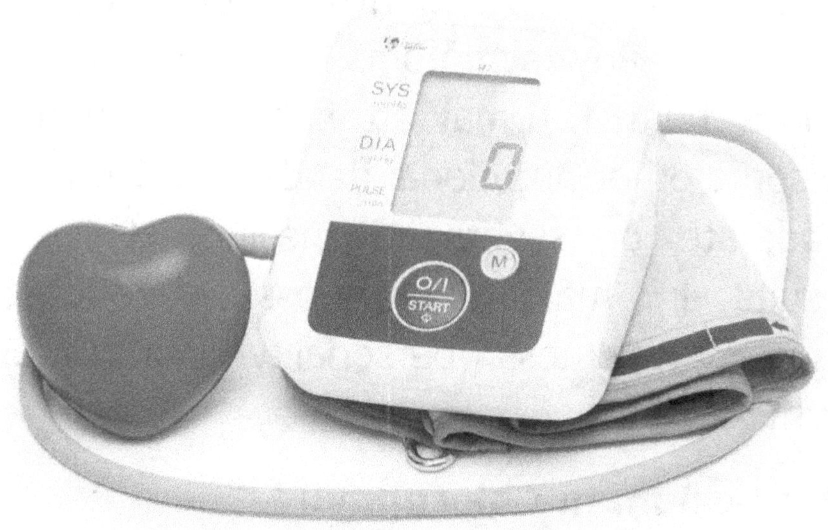

Magnesium the Forgotten Mineral

Half of the magnesium you have in your body is found in your bones and the other half is in your soft tissue. It is found in your skeletal muscles, liver, heart, and pancreas.

Magnesium is considered a "forgotten mineral." Most people don't think about magnesium like they do calcium, potassium or iron. Almost 90% of the population may be short on magnesium since it has been found that they only consume about 40% of the daily recommended requirement.

If you are short in magnesium, you may not show any symptoms or you may just ignore them. You may attribute the symptoms to some other nutritional deficiency. However, moderate or severe magnesium deficiency results in malnutrition, loss of appetite, nausea, weakness, personality changes and arrhythmias.

Magnesium in Chlorophyll

Magnesium is a major mineral like sodium, calcium, and potassium. It is central to the food chain in that it holds a position in chlorophyll, the blood of plants. It appears in the center of the chlorophyll molecule. Chlorophyll is similar to the hemoglobin molecule except that at the center of the hemoglobin molecule is the mineral iron.

So, if you want to build your blood, drinking chlorophyll is one way to do. It's the magnesium in the chlorophyll that also helps make white blood cells that fight infection and which combines with red blood cells.

When your body is low in hemoglobin, drinking chlorophyll will help increase the hemoglobin in your blood. Your body has the power to transmute or to transform magnesium into iron, which helps to make more hemoglobin. It does this through multiple chemical changes that start with oxygen.

Magnesium Requirements

The overall balance of minerals in your body's lymph liquids, outside your cells, and inside your cells, determines your health. When your minerals are balanced similar to seawater, you will have better health.

The sea has a high level of magnesium, so that water inside your cells should also be high in magnesium since magnesium is used to transport nutrients in and out of your cells. Magnesium is a major mineral that is needed in the right quantities so that you can achieve maximum health.

Most people ignore the importance of magnesium. It is important to know what magnesium does in your body. You need to know what foods to eat to get the maximum magnesium in your body. You should know what symptoms you will have when you don't get the proper amount of magnesium.

If you know how magnesium is regulated in your body, then you can help your body maintain and keep the amount that your body needs. Also, if you know what illnesses need more magnesium, you can help yourself get well.

Magnesium and Enzymes

Magnesium is involved in activating over 300 different enzymes and body chemicals. It helps to activate the B vitamins. It works in protein synthesis, muscle excitability and helps to release energy. In your cells, it converts fats, carbohydrates, and protein into energy your body needs. It helps to regulate blood sugar, nerve impulses, and an electrical potential across cell walls. And, it tones brain blood vessels and keeps them relaxed and open, so that nutrients can get into your brain cells.

Magnesium and Bones

You will find magnesium mostly in your cells, in the mitochondria, which is the energy center of your cells. Magnesium regulated the absorption of calcium and maintains the construction of bones and teeth. Lack of magnesium can lead to brittle bones and osteoporosis. Your parathyroid gland also needs magnesium to regulate your blood calcium levels.

Magnesium is the third most important nutrient in building bones, after calcium and vitamin D. Half of all the magnesium in your body is found in your bones. When you lack magnesium, you are susceptible to forming calcium crystals in your bones and in other body locations.

Stress

If you are constantly under stress because of your job, your home life, or your regular life, then most likely, you will be low on magnesium. The same holds true if you stress your body physically by doing exercise and playing sports.

8: How Magnesium Keeps You Disease Free

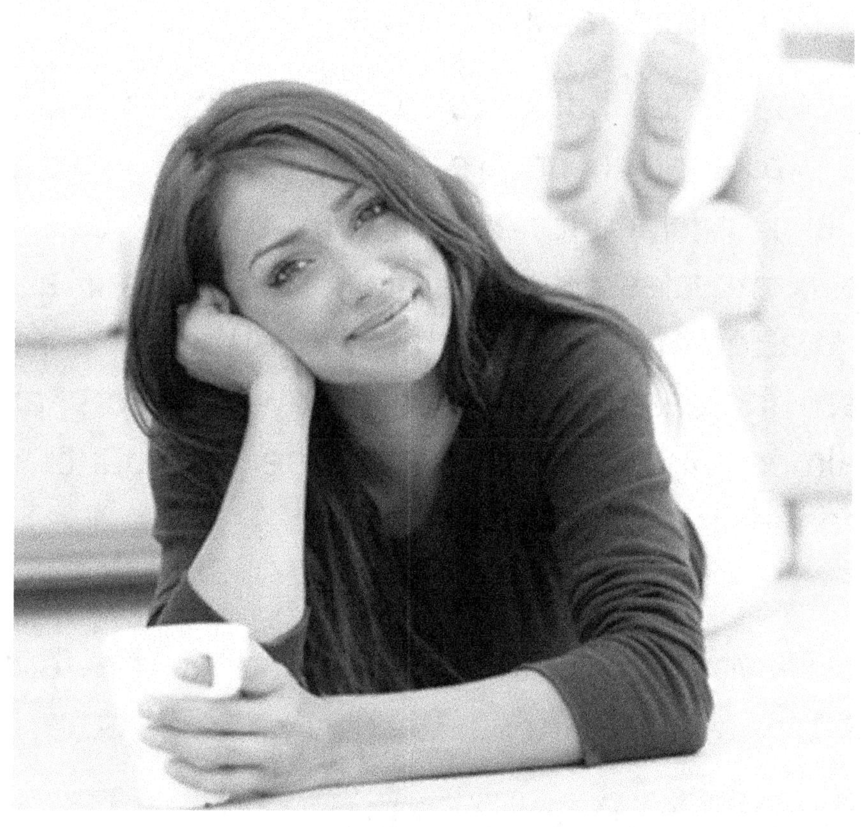

"A mineral that relaxes the body – magnesium"

Like sodium, calcium, and potassium,

magnesium also has a positive charge and is represented by the symbol, Mg+. Because of this, magnesium helps to make your body more alkaline. Your bones hold up to 60% of the body's magnesium, and the extracellular liquid contains around 1%.

Your body holds up to 3 oz. of magnesium. It is alkaline in nature and it is known as the "Relaxer" since it helps to calm the nerves and relax muscles. But, calming the nerves is also a matter of mind control and attitude. You can increase your lifespan when you are calmer and have the proper amount of magnesium in your body.

In your body, magnesium takes the form of:

- Magnesium carbonate
- Magnesium silicate
- Magnesium chloride
- Magnesium sulfate (Epsom salt)
- Magnesium phosphate.

Your body, you have good movement and can do When you have plenty of magnesium in many physical activities. Here is a list of what magnesium does in your body.

- Alkalinizes the body
- Produces laxative action
- Calms the nerves
- Keeps the body flexible
- Influences glands
- Combats acids and toxins
- Eliminates poisons
- Prevents deposition of phosphates in joints
- Neutralizes phosphoric acid
- Promotes carbohydrate metabolism in the cells
- Helps produce and use body energy
- Helps in DNA and protein creation
- Assists Potassium and sodium cross cell membrane during Potassium – Sodium Pump action
- Regulates muscle movements
- Helps maintain calcium levels in the extracellular fluid

Magnesium does its work by reducing

tension, relaxing your body, and improving bowel movements. It reduces nerve irritation when you have excess stress.

Your body regulates the amount of magnesium it retains and stores by using the gastrointestinal tract, GI tract, and urinary system. If you need more magnesium in your body, the GI tract will absorb more in the small intestine. If your body has too much magnesium, the GI tract will excrete some of it and eliminate it through your stools.

Your kidneys are also involved in controlling the amount of magnesium your body retains.

If magnesium levels fall, the kidneys closely control how much magnesium goes into your urine. Similarly, if the magnesium levels are too high, the kidneys will excrete more through your urine.

Regulation of Magnesium

Many things control how much magnesium and calcium you absorb. If magnesium in your body goes up, calcium stores will go down and if magnesium stores fall, then calcium body stores go up. Your stomach absorbs a lot of magnesium for hydrochloric acid production, HCl. When you take in food or calcium supplements, protein, vitamin D, or alcohol, your body needs more magnesium. And, caffeine, sugar, phosphorus, excess sodium, diuretics, and alcohol increase the loss of magnesium through urine.

You will increase the amount of magnesium you absorb, when you drink milk, because of the presence of lactose.

Magnesium as a laxative

Magnesium has natural laxative powers. When you eat foods that have magnesium your regularity improves. When magnesium is consumed and reaches your blood, some of it is transported into your colon walls. Where it softens your stools and helps to produce peristaltic action. For this reason fruits and vegetables that contain some or are high in magnesium promote regularity. Yellow produce such as winter squashes, grapefruits, apricots, oranges, and peaches improve regularity.

Magnesium Supplements

The best magnesium supplements to use are:

- Magnesium citrate
- Magnesium threonate

9: Best Magnesium Foods to Eat Every Day

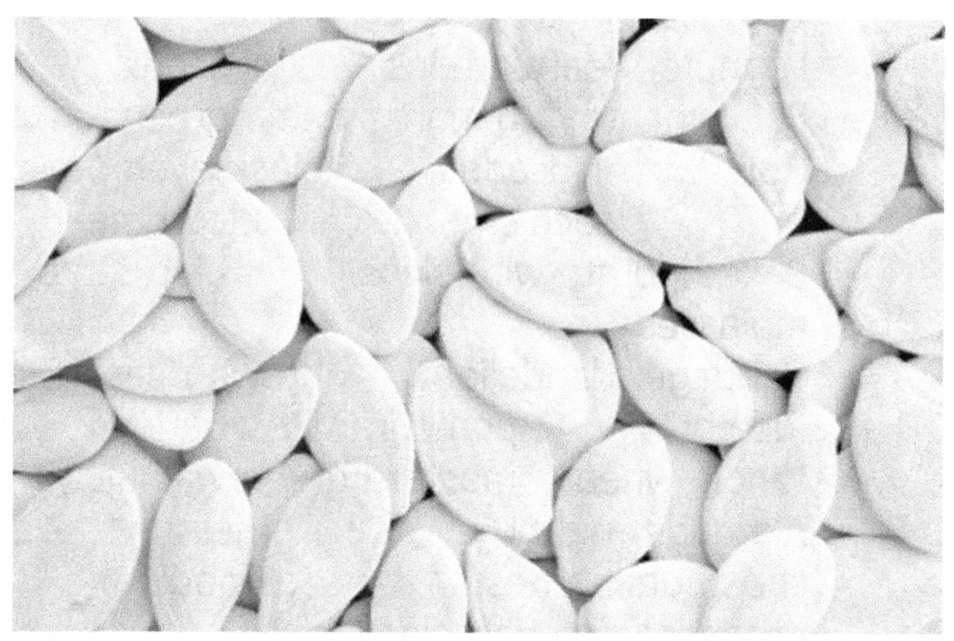

Best Foods with Magnesium

Here is a list of the foods that you should eat to get plenty of magnesium:

Rice bran, pumpkin seeds, wheat germ, sunflower seeds, sesame seeds, seaweed agar, cashews, hazelnuts, fermented soy products

Other great foods for magnesium:

- Peanuts   leafy greens   seeds
- Buckwheat   bananas beet   greens
- Oats   avocados   black-eyed peas   cocoa   cornmeal
- Baked potato with skins   blackstrap molasses
- Cabbage, dandelion   brown rice
- Rice bran,   pomegranates barley
- Whole wheat   mustard green walnut
- Almonds   nuts rye   Nettles
- chestnuts berries   Seafood
- green leafy vegetables
- Dry beans and peas   meat

Chocolate

Many people crave chocolate. This may be because they are deficient in magnesium. Chocolate, especially cocoa, has a high concentration of magnesium. In one cup of unsweetened cocoa, you have 400 mg of magnesium and 2159 mg of potassium. It also has many other minerals but in smaller quantity. Cocoa is also known for its high level of antioxidants.

To get the best benefits of cocoa, you need to eat chocolate that has at least 70% to 85% cocoa.

However, when you eat chocolate candy, which has bittersweet chocolate, or semisweet baking chocolate, it has up to 65% sugar and a fat level of 20 – 35%. Cocoa has 2% sugar and has a fat level of up to 15%. Using unsweetened or bittersweet chocolate in cooking is ok since its sugar level is 2 – 45%. Look for the low sugar products.

What is not good about chocolate is it is also high in caffeine and theobromine, which stimulate the adrenals that can lead to adrenal fatigue.

Yellow Cornmeal

Yellow cornmeal, high in magnesium, has excellent laxative powers. Use it 3 or 4 times a week to improve your regularity. Cornmeal, cooked slowly under low heat, can easily be used with children or adults that are constipated. Or, you can prepare raw corn soup by:

- 1 ½ cups raw corn off the cob

- Vegetable broth to taste

- 2 bay leaves

- 1 ½ cup of raw milk, cream, or milk

- Put all this into a blender and warm slightly

Calms the nerves

Magnesium is a relaxer of nerves. When you are tense, nervous, get irritated, or turn hot-tempered, you develop ulcers, colitis, constipation, and colon spastic conditions.

Magnesium will help to reduce or minimize these conditions. It enters the nerve fibers, with the help of albumin and water.

When you first take magnesium for nerves or for any other condition, you will have to use it for a month or more to see results. It takes that long and even longer for magnesium to fill your body reserves so that it is available to constantly serve your body's needs.

If you have lower back problems, you need to have plenty of magnesium. When you are tense, any adjustments a chiropractor gives will go out of adjustment, when your body is low in magnesium. The adjustment will be made and your tense ligaments or muscles will pull back the adjustment to its previous position.

Magnesium is found in tendons, ligaments, tissue, joints, and nerves and helps them to relax and to maintain bones in position.

Cramps in your calves, at night, call for magnesium and calcium, which prevents the stiffening of tissue and muscle due to excess acids.

Alkalizes the body

Magnesium combines with acids, gases, waste, impurities, and toxins to clean your body and make your body more alkaline. Magnesium sulfate pulls toxic buildup and waste from your intestinal walls and eliminates them through your stools.

A good supply of magnesium is necessary to make your body alkaline and to combine with poisons and heavy metals. Magnesium has the ability to combine with poisons that create diseases. It combines with excess albumin, lead, phosphorus, chloride, antimony, ferrous sulfate, barium, muriatic acid, uric acid, urate acid, and ptomaine.

In the brain, magnesium combines with phosphoric by-products that occur when you do excessive mental work.

10: Deficiency And Excesses Of Magnesium

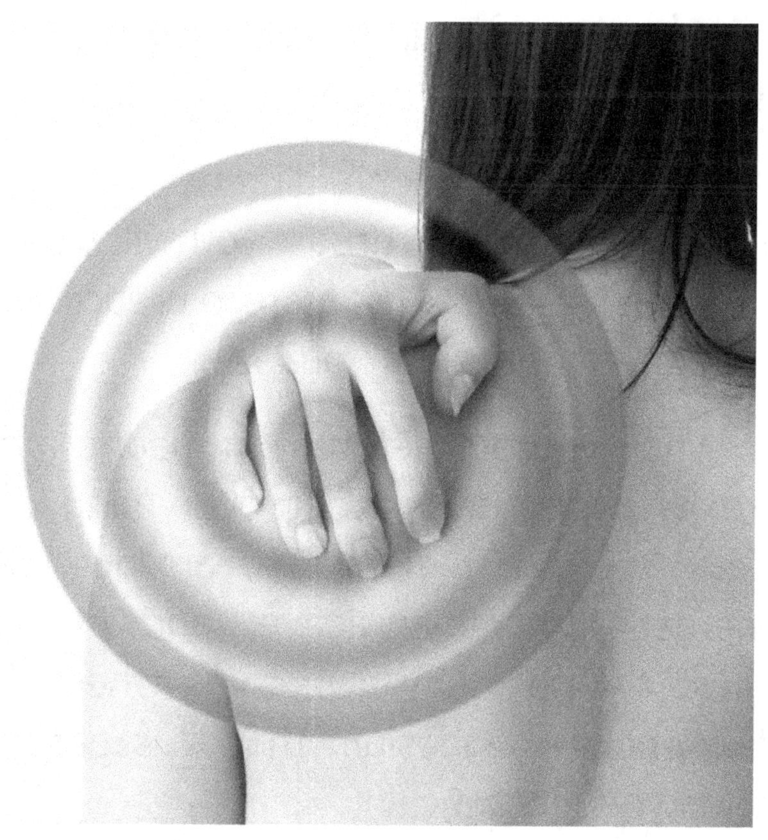

Deficiencies of Magnesium

When you become dehydrated, you lose magnesium. When you take calcium you will deplete your stores of magnesium. Drinking too much milk also will deplete your body's magnesium.

Young athletes that drink too much milk need to be careful since they tend to lose magnesium. Retired and geriatric people should always take a magnesium supplement.

If you are taking diuretics of any kind, natural remedies or drugs, you will slowly lose your magnesium. The more diuretics you use the more magnesium you lose.

When you are deficient in magnesium, you are over sensitive about everything in your life. You are hyperactive, anxious, fidgety, energetic, mentally active, and industrious. There are so many symptoms when you are deficient in magnesium that it is hard to tell when you are deficient.

The more serious symptoms are muscle spasms and seizures. There is now some evidence that magnesium deficiency has an important role in many heart ailments. Dr.

Alexander Heggtveit, at the University of Ottawa in Canada, found fatal attack victims with less magnesium than those that died of other causes.

You can have a magnesium deficiency after prolonged diarrhea and vomiting or with long-term laxative and diuretic use. If you frequently drink too much alcohol then, you will be deficient in magnesium.

Elderly people are at high risk for magnesium deficiency since they absorb it poorly. If they supplement with too much calcium or use too many drugs, this can deplete their magnesium body stores.

When you have a low level of magnesium, you will have an increase in calcium blood levels, which contribute to the formation of kidney stones. If the low levels continue, magnesium will be pulled out of the heart muscles, causing a disruption in its function.

When your blood levels of magnesium are low, your body takes magnesium that is stored in your tissues, which leads to muscle weakness, fatigue, irritability, and nervousness.

Here is a list of symptoms you can have when you have a low level of magnesium.

- Head tremors
- Voice breaks or stammers
- Unclear conversations
- Feeling of doom
- Smelly feet
- Muscles are weak
- Constipation
- Poor kidney function
- Poor sleep
- Back pain
- Heart palpitations
- Eyelids twitch
- Osteoporosis
- High blood pressure
- Migraine headaches
- Appetite for acid food and drink
- Nausea
- Heavy head in the morning
- Shoulder and neck muscles tense at night

Hypomagnesemia

A deficiency in magnesium is called Hypomagnesemia. This deficiency is when the amount of your body's magnesium falls below 1.8mEq/L. The unit mEq/L is a measure given to the amount of substance in a body per liter. This deficiency can occur when you:

- don't eat enough magnesium foods
- have poor absorption of magnesium in GI tract
- have excess magnesium loss in GI tract
- have excess magnesium loss in urinary tract – kidney
- use excess coffee, alcohol, sugar, and tobacco

Negative emotions also deplete magnesium that is in reserves and in intracellular liquid. If you constantly live these emotions below, then you will be short of magnesium:

Hatred, resentment, jealousy, quarrels, bitterness, temper outbursts, selfishness, greed, fear, panic, worry, paranoia, overwork, over study, loss of loved one.

Other symptoms you can have with low magnesium are:

- Cardiac arrhythmias
- Digoxin toxicity
- Laryngeal strid or Respiratory muscle weakness
- Seizures
- Arthritis deformations
- Poor elimination
- Over-excitement
- Nervous headaches
- Ulcers
- Acute diarrhea
- Eyes tearing excessively or excess catarrh of the eye lens
- Nosebleeds
- Sex brain nerve ends and nerve fiber irritation
- Decrease in electrical nerve impulses
- Extreme colitis
- Urine retention
- Sleeplessness, fainting
- Hot temper, forgetfulness
- Drastic mood changes

- Increase in asthmatic attacks
- Free Radical Damage

When you are magnesium deficient, the body starts taking magnesium out of your cells. As you reduce cell magnesium, your muscles grow weak and nerves and muscles become highly irritable.

Free Radical Damage

Low levels of magnesium can magnify the damage caused by free radicals. It has also been seen that it can start the production of free radicals.

Excess of Magnesium

You can have excess magnesium in your body when you eat an excess of magnesium foods, supplements, tonics or drugs. When you have an excess of magnesium in your body, the sedative effects of magnesium are intensified. Your memory decreases, you become less active and do not have good reasoning skills. Your nerve endings become less sensitive and depressed and your perception and intelligence are decreased. You become less interested in life and you sleep more.

Hypermagnesemia

Excessive magnesium in your body is called Hypermagnesemia. This condition occurs when you have a magnesium level above 2.5 mEq/L. This condition is rare since kidneys can quickly remove excess magnesium. But, when it does occur, and the cause could be:

- Kidney dysfunction
- Addison's disease
- Adrenocortical insufficiency
- Excess use of antacids or laxatives
- Excess use of magnesium-rich dialysate
- Excess use of TPN solutions
- Excess use of magnesium sulfate in treating seizures, or hypertension

Patellar Reflex

If your patellar reflex, the tapping just below the knee to see if the leg extension occurs, is absent, it's an indication that your magnesium level is 7 mEq/L or higher. This high level makes your nerves relax creating an absence of leg reflex in the patellar test.

Magnesium Laxative

Excess magnesium is quickly removed, from your body by the onset of diarrhea. But, one of the issues is that you can develop an excess of magnesium when you use a large amount over-the-counter, drugstore products, for acid reflux or constipation. Overdose of magnesium is a rare occurrence.

Large amounts of magnesium can be toxic. You can end up with excess magnesium, if you have kidney disease or if your calcium body levels are low and your phosphorus intake is high.

11: The Best Magnesium Supplements to Use

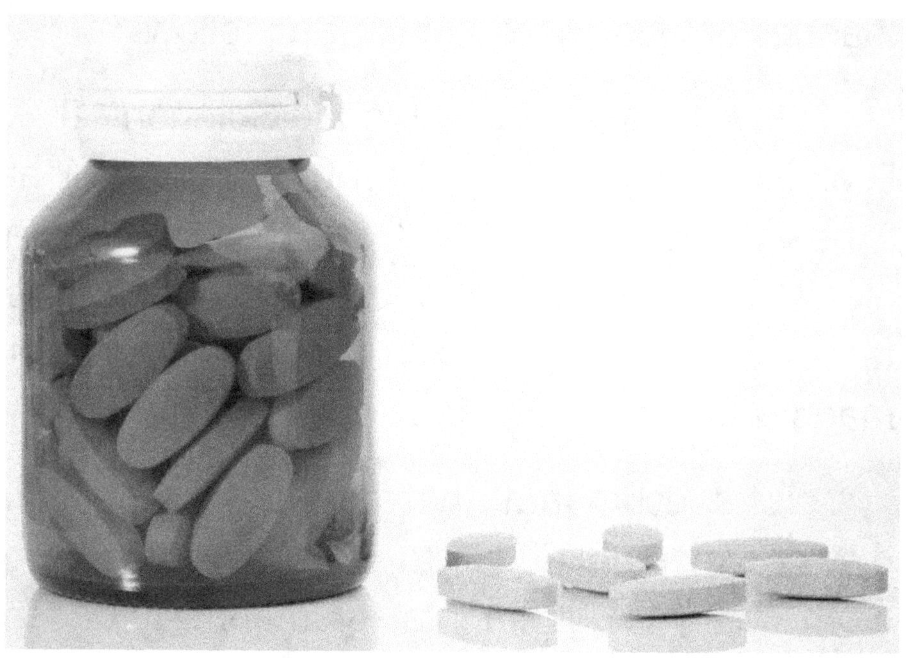

Taking Magnesium Supplements

Do not take magnesium supplements if you have kidney weakness or disease. Also, if you have heart problems, do not take more than 350 mg of magnesium. It is always safe to see your doctor about what dose you should take.

Fast Magnesium

If you have gut spasms or other body conditions where you need to receive magnesium fast, you can do it as follows:

Buy a Magnesium Chloride Solution 18%, Ecologic Formulas Brand, on the internet or at a health food store. Add 1-2 teaspoons to a glass of water and drink twice a day. The taste is not too good, but you will get magnesium into your body quickly.

It is estimated that a typical American diet provides only 30% to 50% of the 500 mg of the daily requirements for magnesium. In addition, around 80% of the diets eaten in American are magnesium deficient.

Magnesium is easier to lose than other minerals and especially when you eat or take an increase in calcium. When you supplement with magnesium you should check that the supplement has equal amounts of magnesium and calcium. If it has more calcium, you will lose some magnesium. Or, it would be better to take magnesium as a separate supplement and taken when you don't take calcium.

Magnesium Citrate

Use a magnesium citrate supplement. Take this supplement after 8 pm with vitamin C and pantothenic acid, since these three nutrients work together. Always take magnesium and all other minerals and trace minerals with tomato juice or apple juice or at meals with whole grapes, meat or digestive enzymes.

This provides acid to dissolve and absorb the magnesium quicker. You can also take it after 8 pm or just before bedtime without any food.

There are other forms of magnesium that are also good since they are tied to an amino acid or are so-called "chelated." These are,

- Magnesium citrate
- Magnesium gluconate,

- Magnesium Aspartate
- Magnesium taurate
- Magnesium oxide – avoid using this type, because it is not as absorbable as the other types.

Magnesium and Calcium Supplements

Look for a combination supplement of calcium, magnesium, vitamin D, vitamin, K2 and with a 1:1 ratio of calcium to magnesium. This type of ratio is hard to find, but, you should be able to find it on the internet. Most ratios you will find are 2:1 with calcium being twice as much as magnesium.

Here are other magnesium combinations that you should consider if you can't find the supplements above:

Potassium- magnesium citrate

Magnesium citrate – potassium- taurine

Magnesium can interfere with any antibiotic you might be taking, so it best not to supplement with it when taking antibiotics or even other drugs.

How Much Magnesium?

Some doctors and nutritionists say that you should have twice as much magnesium as calcium in your supplement. This will ensure that you will have strong bones. Most supplements that contain these minerals are of the opposite ratio; they have twice as much calcium as magnesium. But, taking a supplement with a 1:1 ratio should be where you can start.

Daily magnesium supplementation is:

- Children to 14 years, 270 mg

- Males 15 and older, 500 mg

- Males 51 years and older 600 mg

- Females 15 and older, 300 mg

- Females 51 years and older 550 mg

In some cases for adults, up to 1200 mg is recommended. Overdosing is very hard with magnesium since the kidney and the colon will excrete the excess. If you start to exhibit signs of diarrhea or body weakness, back off on the amount you are taking.

Vitamin D

You need the proper levels of magnesium to activate the vitamin D your body needs. If you have a magnesium deficiency, then you will have lower levels of vitamin D. Make sure, you use the Vitamin D3 type of supplement.

B vitamins

When you take Vitamin B6, you improve the intake of magnesium into your cells. You can supplement with a vitamin B 50 or 100 to get the needed B vitamins.

Copper

Because magnesium is easily lost in the urine, when you are dehydrated, you can take 3 mg of copper and this will stop the loss of magnesium in your urine.

Over The Counter Magnesium Products

Magnesium toxicity can occur in individuals with kidney failure. Toxicity effects have been found in some individuals that use laxatives such as Epsom salts, magnesium sulfate and milk of magnesia, or magnesium hydroxide. These laxatives are typically used at 3,000 to 5,000 mg per day. Toxic effects have been found when these laxatives are used at 9,000 mg per day.

If you have a deficiency of magnesium, it will take around 6 months of magnesium supplementation to get your body back to normal levels of magnesium. Your body uses magnesium every day, so you need to supply it with magnesium every day. Any excess can go to neutralize acids. Then if still have some left over, this will go to various body areas to be stored.

12: Illnesses Magnesium Eliminates

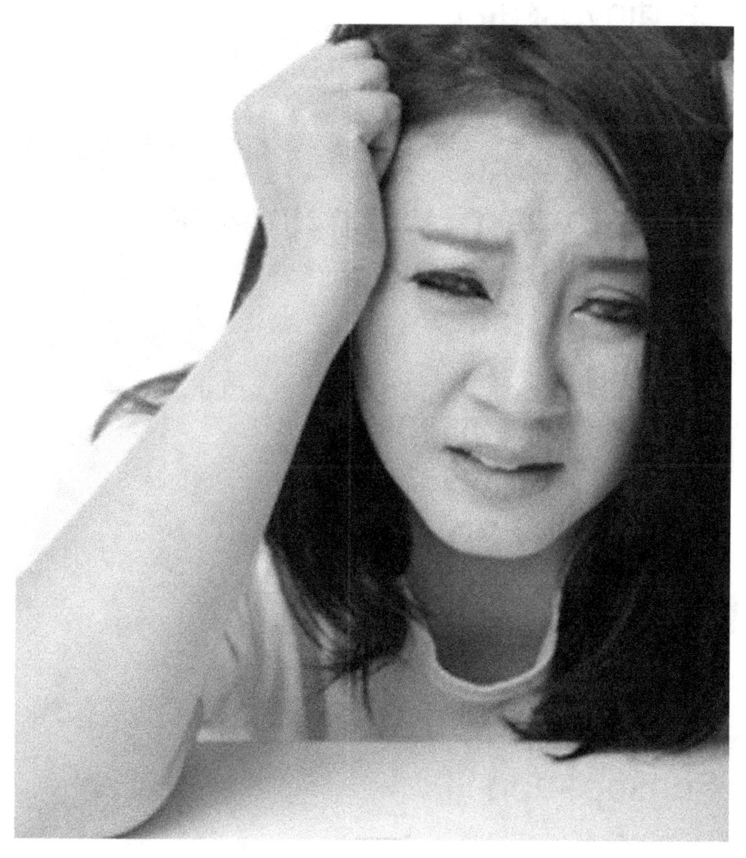

There are certain illnesses that you can reduce, eliminate and even cure if you increase your intake of magnesium. Some of these illnesses are caused by the lack of magnesium.

These illnesses are:

- Cardiovascular
- Chronic fatigue syndrome
- Kidney stones
- Muscle cramps
- Preeclampsia – during pregnancy
- Osteoporosis
- PMS symptoms
- Migraines
- Respiratory disease
- Alzheimer's disease
- Back problems
- Free Radicals
- Migraines
- Digestive Problems
- Eye problems
- Constipation

Cardiovascular

Having a low level of magnesium can result in more blood clots.

It has been found that women that use oral contraceptive have lower levels of magnesium. This is the reason why there is a higher occurrence of thrombosis in women that use these contraceptives.

A deficiency of magnesium can damage the arteries in the heart, which results in plaque buildup. High blood pressure is also associated with a magnesium deficiency. There is a tendency for those with diabetes and low magnesium to have more cardiovascular issues.

So keep your levels of magnesium high by eating and supplementing with the suggestions given here. Magnesium helps to reduce the possibility of you having a heart attack, stroke, angina, or heart surgery. Eating nuts of various kinds every workday will help you stop heart attacks.

Kidney Stones

If you have kidney stones, you can get rid of them by using 1000 mg of magnesium citrate and 100 mg of B6. If you just want to make sure you don't accumulate stones, you can use this supplement combination on occasion for a week. Kidney stones are a combination of calcium and oxalic acid. When these two combine in the kidney they form calcium oxalate crystals.

To minimize the amount of oxalic acid you have in your body, avoid eating cooked spinach or other green tops. Eat them raw when possible.

Muscle Cramps

Magnesium helps to relax the muscle and without it, you are prone to muscle cramps. When calcium moves into muscle tissue, your muscles will contract. When calcium leaves the muscles, and magnesium moves into your muscles, your muscles will relax. Excess deficiency of magnesium leads to muscle spasms, tremors, and convulsions. If you have leg cramps at night, take a combination of calcium, magnesium, and vitamin D. This will put an end to these cramps. Take this supplement just before bedtime.

Osteoporosis

To have strong bones and teeth you need minerals. It's calcium that makes bones strong in conjunction with other minerals such as phosphorous, magnesium, strontium, silica, zinc, copper, and boron. Magnesium is definitely needed to prevent osteoporosis.

PMS symptoms

There are some women that crave chocolate before their period or who have PMS. It is known that magnesium helps resolve the symptoms of PMS since it is involved in the production of progesterone. A lack of magnesium can produce less progesterone levels resulting in PMS symptoms.

It's better to avoid chocolate since it creates adrenal fatigue. It is better to eat those foods that are high in magnesium or to take 400 mg of magnesium citrate. Take this magnesium with some vitamin C and B6 just before bedtime.   Magnesium is absorbed better after 8 pm. This combination of nutrients will help to reduce the intensity and duration of PMS.

Pregnancy

Magnesium has a powerful influence in the prevention of pregnancy complication, such as prematurity and intrauterine growth retardation.

Migraines

There are studies that show magnesium can prevent or relieve migraines. By using high doses of 1000 mg or more, magnesium was shown to be just as effective as established drugs, such as flunarizine and amitriptyline.

Respiratory Disease

Magnesium has been found to be helpful in respiratory diseases such as bronchitis and asthma. Eat those foods that are high in magnesium, but you need to be aware of those foods that you might be allergic to, which aggravate your respiratory condition.

Alzheimer's Disease

Having a low level of magnesium and calcium in your body opens you up to toxic aluminum deposit in your brain nerve cells. When you have a low level of these minerals, your body will accept the use of other minerals in their place. So, if you also have an excess of aluminum, your body will use it in place of magnesium or calcium and when these minerals reach your brain they deposit in your brain cells.

If aluminum continues to accumulate in brain amyloid, this condition can lead to poor brain function. Under these conditions, zinc is the recommend mineral to prevent senile changes in your brain.

Magnesium is involved in keeping your brain cells alive. It does this by reducing the negative effects of less blood flow to the brain and by ensuring that nutrients reach your brain cells. It also prevents the buildup of calcium in your brain cells, which is associated with Alzheimer's.

Back Problems

Magnesium will help you build a strong straight back. It aids in the inter-vertebral structure. It is in this structure where magnesium is stored. It is also stored in the colon. If the vertebral structure and colon don't get enough magnesium, they will not function properly.

Free Radicals

It has been seen by researchers that low levels of magnesium give way to free radical formation thus exposing cells to more radical attack.

Migraines

It has been found that 50% of people with migraines have a magnesium deficiency. You can get some relief by taking 400+ mg of magnesium daily with meals.

Digestive Problems

If you have stomach problems such as vomiting, cramps, indigestion, flatulence, stomach pain, or constipation, all of this could be related to low levels of magnesium

Eye problems

If you are diabetic, you will want to keep high levels of blood magnesium. If you do, you are less likely to develop diabetic retinopathy. In addition, if you have glaucoma, it will lessen the effects of this condition.

Constipation

Magnesium is hydrophilic and likes water. In your colon, it will draw water and make your stools soft. Magnesium is used in many over-the-counter laxatives. Using these laxatives give you high levels of magnesium salts. If you are deficient in magnesium, you will have constipation.

Sweaty Hands

Have you ever shaken hands with someone that has sweaty hands or that has excess body odor? Aside from not showering frequently, this person may be deficient in magnesium. The use of liquid chlorophyll will help reduce body odor.

13: Final Tips on Using Magnesium

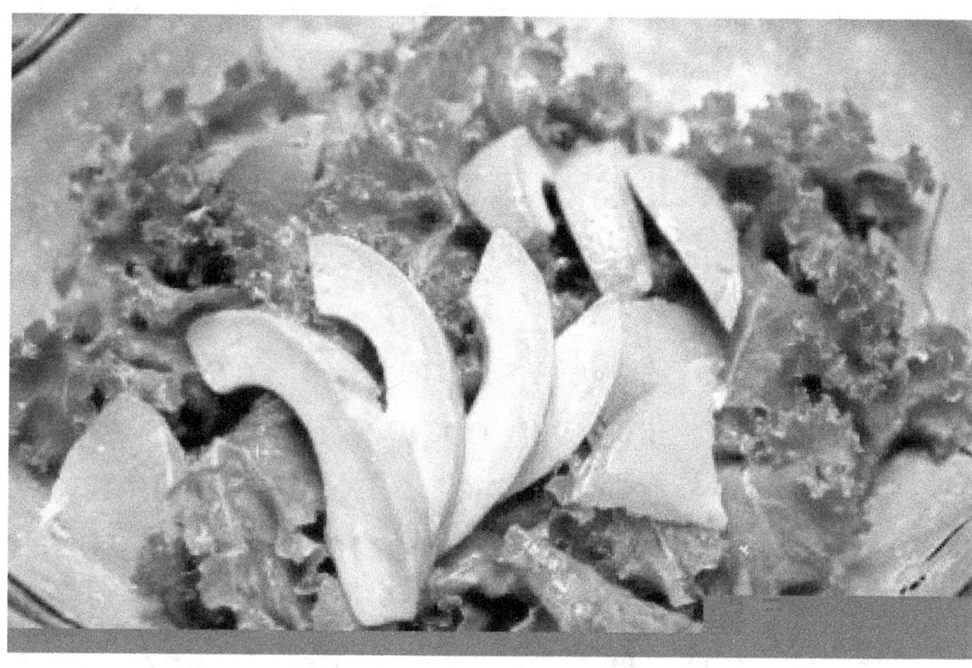

In your cells, tissues, muscles, and nerves, magnesium neutralizes acids, toxic matter, and wastes that are created when you become anxious, nervous, hot-tempered, overexcited, or overworked. It helps to neutralize those acids that come from eating too much acid food. Use magnesium foods and supplements to help get your body alkaline.

When you eat a lot of meat and other acid foods with little vegetables, you will deplete your stores of magnesium and you will need to use all the information listed in this book to restore your magnesium body levels. Magnesium is known as the "Relaxer" since it calms your nervous and muscular system.

You can have an under or oversupply of magnesium in your body. Your kidney and colon are responsible for maintaining the proper magnesium balance in your body. It will excrete excessive magnesium into your urine or it will stop excreting it when your body supplies are low. And, with under supplies, magnesium will be pulled out of your cells to satisfy your body's needs. When it does this your body will be acidic and prone to disease.

Eat Magnesium Foods

Eat magnesium foods daily. Use seeds in your smoothies and nuts as midday snacks. Eat a variety of vegetables. Choosing 4 or 5 vegetable properly can give you plenty of all the minerals you need. However, by choosing a variety of fruits and vegetables, you get certain nutrients and antioxidants that are only available in each fruit or vegetable.

Magnesium Supplements

When you buy a magnesium supplement it is best to buy it with calcium and vitamin D3. Calcium needs magnesium and vitamin D3 to complete its digestion and absorption into your body. Choose those supplements that are tied to an amino acid, like Magnesium Citrate. This allows this mineral to be pulled through your intestinal wall easier and faster. Look for a magnesium supplement that has just as much magnesium as calcium, 1:1.

If you have a lot of anxiety and stress in your life you will need to take up to 1000 mg of magnesium. Stress uses up a lot of magnesium.

Look at the list of illnesses and body conditions listed in the previous chapters and see if you have some of these symptoms or diseases. If so, then you too should be taking up to 1000 mg of magnesium. If you have issues with your kidney or heart, then talk to your doctor about how much magnesium you should take.

Excess Magnesium

If you take too much magnesium, you will get diarrhea. Just back off on the amount you are taking, until your diarrhea goes away.

14: The Best Way to Use Ca, Mg, K, and D3

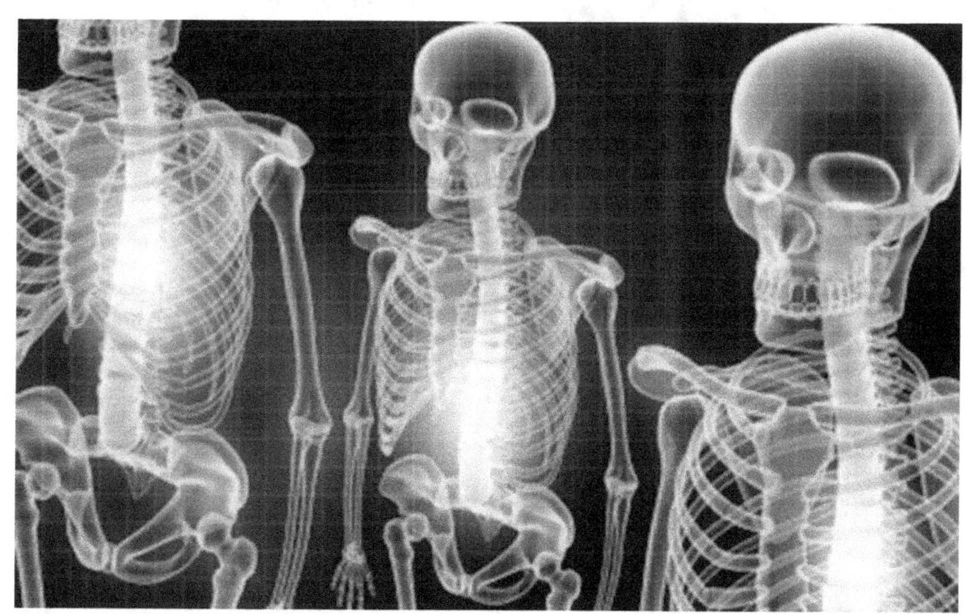

Vitamin D3, the Hormone

Vitamin D3 is considered a hormone and not a vitamin. It was mislabeled a vitamin, during the time it was discovered, since it was thought to come from food. The vitamin form that is active in your body is Vitamin D3, known as cholecalciferol. Vitamin D3 is tasked with communicating with your DNA. It turns on and off over 1000 genes to activate their function.

There is also vitamin D2, which is considerably less active in your body. D3 is around 300% more active in your body than D2. Most foods that are fortified with vitamin D use the D2 form.

Vitamin D3 is created when UV light activates a conversion form of cholesterol, which occurs in or on your skin.

D3 Helps Absorb Calcium

Another vitamin D3 function is to help you absorb calcium. Calcium aside from helping to form bone structures is a key mineral in helping to keep your body alkaline. An alkaline body is the natural state of your body, and an acid body is a state of disease. You can gain more information on how to maintain an alkaline body in my ebook called **"Alkaline Body"**

How Much Vitamin D3 do You Need?

So, what is the dose for vitamin D3? During the 30's and 40's studies showed that taking more than 50,000 IU was still safe. However, pharmaceuticals went on a scare tactic by saying that taking more than 400 IU of vitamin D was toxic.

Yet, being out in the sun for 30 minutes can produce 10,000 to 20,000 IU of vitamin D3.

When vitamin D3 was demonized during the 40's, the pharmaceuticals came out with three miracle drugs for treating various deadly diseases. These drugs were nothing more than 50,000 IU of vitamin D.

The amount of vitamin D3 you may need will depend on a couple of factors. The more obese you are the more D3 you need. You can experiment on how much you need by seeing what result you get with different doses. Take a certain amount in 3 to 4 weeks to see if your health improves.

You can start as follows:

- Normal weight – 5,000 to 10,000 IU

- Overweight – 8,000 to 12,000

- Obese – 8,000 to 15,000

If you take over 10,000 IU of vitamin D3, you will have to supplement with vitamin 1000 mcg of K2 to avoid calcium depositing in body tissue and joints.

You should be ok to take up and more than 20,000 IU of vitamin D3. To do this you must take a minimum of 1000 mcg of vitamin K2 per 10,000 IU of vitamin D3. Be sure not to take too much K2, since it can cause a racing heart or high blood pressure. If this happens, you would then just back off on the K2, until those symptoms disappear.

Doses of 8,000 IU, in studies, did not

exhibit excess calcium in the blood. The additional calcium brought into the blood by high D3 supplementation, was found to be properly used by the body.

Because D3 is fat soluble, you can optimize its adsorption by taking a healthy fat with it.

Calcium, Vitamin D3, and K2

Vitamin D3 helps to move calcium passed your small intestinal barrier and into your blood. Vitamin K2 then moves the calcium to the right areas of your body. K2 prevents calcium from building up along your arteries and accumulating in your soft tissue and bones. Recent studies show that K2 is beneficial in the treatment of rheumatoid arthritis. K2 is also known improving blood clotting.

Types of Vitamin K

There are several kinds of vitamin K. There

are K1 and K2, where K2 has several forms of which K7 is the most active and important form. K2 (MK-4) has also shown to be beneficial for rheumatoid arthritis, RA. However, since K7 is more bioavailable then MK-4, it is the better choice for treating RA.

Aside from vitamin D3 being necessary for proper calcium absorption, strong bones, teeth, immune system, heart health, it is also useful in the prevention of cancer and other diseases. Low levels of Vitamin D3 are associated with most every disease you develop.

In the NaturalHealth365 website article, Lori Alton, staff writer, writes,

"According to the Institute of Medicine, 4,000 IU daily is the tolerable upper level of intake – defined as the highest level that would be unlikely to cause harm to nearly all adults. However, the Vitamin D Council recommends that adults take 5,000 IU of the vitamin a day.

Meanwhile, a naturopathic practitioner might advise dosages in the area of 8,000 IU of vitamin D a day, depending on the individual's history and lifestyle. The Endocrine Society Practice Guidelines maintain that adults can safely take up to 10,000 IU a day – more than double what the IOM advises as the safe upper level.

Bottom line: ensuring that you have adequate levels of vitamin D3 just might be one of the most important things you can do to protect your health – and your life."

The supplement to take is one that has calcium, magnesium, vitamin D3, and vitamin K. If you can't find such a supplement, build one from single nutrients. To enhance the effectiveness of vitamin D3, take fish or coconut oil pill.

Alzheimer's' Disease

Low levels of body vitamin D3 have been associated with a higher risk of Alzheimer's' Disease. In addition, other diseases such as cancer (colon, prostate), respiratory infections, multiple sclerosis, and Parkinson's disease have also been associated with low D3 blood levels.

Simply by increasing your blood levels of D3, you give yourself protection against these diseases. Optimum blood levels of D3 are **50 ng/ml to 80 ng/ml**

Respiratory Infections

In a study made at Queen Mary University in London, researchers found that Vitamin D3 was just as effective as getting a flu shot in protecting against a respiratory infection. It was found that Vitamin D3 produces over 210 antimicrobials.

Immune System

It has been discovered that Vitamin D receptors have been found in all immune cells. Further studies show that various autoimmune disorders benefit from increased Vitamin D3 supplementation.

Heart Disease

Low levels of blood vitamin D3 have been associated with cardiovascular and stroke issues. Higher levels of D3 are related to the lowest risks of heart attack, stroke, and death.

Magnesium

Magnesium is necessary for calcium to function properly in your body. It also activates enzymes that help your body use vitamin D3. Without magnesium, vitamin D3 cannot be used by your body. For this reason, it is not a good idea to take calcium without magnesium, vitamin D3, and vitamin K2.

To get many of the other minerals that aid in the proper function of calcium, D3, and K2, eat those foods that are high in magnesium.

You should also supplement with magnesium. The supplements to use are

Nutrients Needed by Vitamin D3

There are many other nutrients that interact with D3. These can come from your diet. Vitamin A, zinc, and boron are few important ones.

Food That Has D3

Very little D3 is found in food. The foods that have some D3 are eggs, wild cold water fish, and organic mushrooms, soy (non GMO), unsweetened yogurt, and ricotta cheese.

Final Words on Vitamin D3

Many studies have been done on vitamin D3 and have substantiated the need to use it in doses up to 10,000 IU or more. The recommended RDA of 400 IU is totally out of line with the body's need for this vitamin, especially if you are sick.

In combination with calcium, magnesium, and K2, vitamin D3 immerges as the nutrient required in large quantities necessary for quality health.

Studies have shown that healthy blood levels of Vitamin D3 are in the range of 50 to 80 ng/ml. Blood level below 30 ng/ml has always shown to be associated with all kinds of disease. The amount of vitamin D3 required for good health has been established to be 5,000 to 10,000 IU of vitamin D3.

Here are the recommended supplement program by Robert R. Barefoot, Nutritionist and BioChemist, as stated in his 2002 book, Death by Diet.

The pH listed below is based on your saliva test listed in this book.

pH	calcium	magnesium	vit. D3	vit. A
6.5 - 7.4	1200mg	690mg	2400IU	30000IU
6.0 - 6.5	2400mg	1380mg	4800IU	60000IU
4.5 - 6.0	3600mg	2070mg	7200IU	90000IU

The pH listed in the above chart is associated with the following body conditions.

pH 6.5 to 7.4 is the normal body condition
pH 6.0 to 6.5 is where the body is developing a disease

pH 4.5 to 6.0 is where you have a disease

Vitamin K

If you take less than 10,000 mg of vitamin D3, you may not need to take any vitamin K. But, if you are taking 10,000 IU or more you should take 1000mcg of K2 with some 100mcg of k7. The k7 is much stronger than the K1 or K2.

Side effects of Vitamin K

Some people have experienced Vitamin K side effects when they have taken too much. These side effects are high blood pressure, headaches, racing heart, and so on. When you experience these side effects, simply back off on the amount of vitamin K you are taking, until the side effect disappear

15: About the Author With Resources

Rudy Silva is a natural consultant nutritionist educated in the United State in Nutrition and Physics. He is a graduate of San Jose State University in California. He is the author of 40 other books on natural remedies. He has authored a newsletter in natural remedies for over 4 years. He has many websites promoting special recommended products and information.

Resource page

Here are some other books on natural remedies that have been written by this author. To see all of his books go to the internet and search on Google, Rudy Silva.

If you need support or want to promote any of his books, please contact him at 24 hours.

He looks forward to hearing from you and is happy to help you understand his material on natural and nutritional health.

Give A Review

And, don't forget to give a review for this book, so that others can gain the benefits of what is in this book.

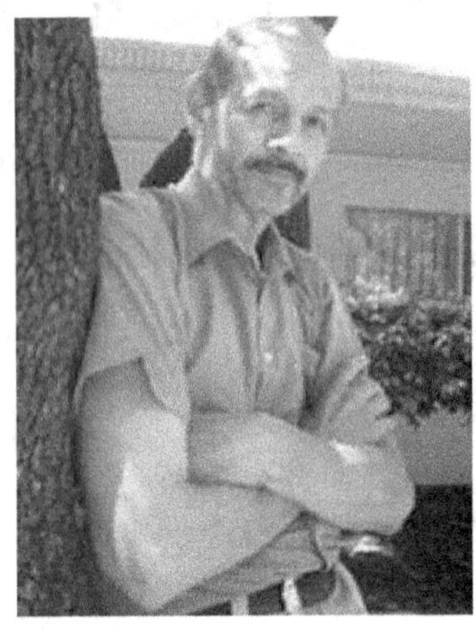

To you, eliminating disease, and creating better health and more happiness in your life,

Rudy S Silva